Tales of a Spoonie Warrior

Chronicles of the Chronically Ill

Saidee Wynn

ISBN: 1718800851
ISBN-13: 978-1718800854

DEDICATION

For Matt, who is more than my rock, he's my mountain. And for Harper, who always inspires me to be better.

CONTENTS

ACKNOWLEDGMENTS

I want to thank all the people who've supported me and all my dreams, no matter how wild and impossible they seemed. In particular, Matt and Harper who put up with all my writer's antics. Rebecca, for editing my musings and putting up with my constant questioning. My dad for always believing in me, and making sure we're always okay. My mom for encouraging me to be keep writing, even when I thought it I wasn't any good. My best friend, Halley, who helped me brainstorm and has always been a great cheerleader. All my other friends and family, who have served as inspirations for my writings far more than they may realize. And, all my readers from spooniewarrior.com. Without all of you, this never would've happened.

INTRODUCTION TO A LIFE INVISIBLE

I'm just gonna go ahead and jump right in here. Hello, I'm Saidee and I have an invisible illness. Multiple actually. Well, they are invisible to most, but they are very visible to me.

I see it in my purple feet, thanks to blood pooling in my legs. I see it in the weight I've gained due to exercise intolerance. I see it in my weekly schedule, high on doctor's appointments and low on social engagements. I see it in the loss of a career I loved greatly. I see it in my daughter's face when I tell her I can't pick her up or carry her. What is invisible to many, is so clearly visible in my life. And being invisible can feel incredibly isolating.

An article on umass.edu states that "It is estimated that 10% of people in the U.S. have a medical condition which could be considered a type of invisible disability." It goes on to estimate that one in two Americans has some type of chronic medical condition. One in two! Half of the US population is walking around with an "invisible" condition and, yet, most of us are walking around feeling completely alone.

An invisible illness, as you've probably guessed, is an illness that isn't immediately visible to others. Such conditions include: depression, anxiety disorder, Ehlers-Danlos syndrome,

SAIDEE WYNN

fibromyalgia, Postural Orthostatic Tachycardia Syndrome, Celiac's disease, Irritable Bowel Syndrome, and so many others that I could never possibly name them all. These conditions range from common to rare.

I happen to have multiple invisible illnesses which have become debilitating for me. When I am in my wheelchair or using my rollator, my illness becomes visible to others. I have run into many people who are quick to help me or accommodate my needs when I am using a medical device. I get looks of pity and am often talked down to, but we'll save that for another chapter. No one second guesses my use of disability parking or needing to rest.

But when I'm out in public without my wheelchair or my rollator, I am met with looks of criticism and judgement. I get eye-rolls that read "God, what a drama queen," if I'm out and exclaim to my husband that I need to sit down so that I won't pass out. I've had people laugh when they hear me out of breath after walking across a parking lot, they don't realize that I'm panting because my heart rate is getting dangerously high and I'm on the verge of passing out. I've heard several whispers and snickers because of my not-so-fashionable compression socks and leggings. I wonder if they would still be whispering and judging me if they knew that my compression wear is the only thing keeping my blood from just sitting in my legs instead of circulating?

How is it that 50% of US citizens have some kind of chronic medical condition, and yet, our society immediately assumes that someone walking slowly is just being a pain in the ass rather than having a legitimate medical condition? Even with my wheelchair, if someone sees me stand up and get out of it, their looks go from pitying (not an enjoyable look either) to horrified and judgmental. There are several different reasons that someone might need a wheelchair. Being paraplegic is only one of them.

Could it be that the reason people have a hard time believing in and understanding invisible illnesses is because they are so often kept hidden? Or is it that we feel we have to

4

hide our illnesses away to make others feel comfortable? Often, as I explain my condition to people, I see their eyes gloss over and their faces contort into an expression that says, "Oh dear god, what do I do? This is so awkward." They seem unsure of how to handle what I'm telling them. Are they supposed to pity me? Are they supposed to offer solutions? Are they supposed to tell me they'll pray for me? Or that they're sure that things will get better one day?

I have heard all of those reactions and more. I end up feeling trapped in this weird place of wondering if I should be honest and talk about what's going on in my life or pretend that everything is ok so that the conversation doesn't get weird. But then, I'm not really left with much to say, because my illnesses are a pretty big part of my life right now. They inform most everything that I do. There isn't a day that goes by where I don't have to think about my health. Leaving out my illnesses in everyday conversation feels like I'm being dishonest because, honestly, they are an everyday thing.

So, I choose to talk about my illnesses. I refuse to stay hidden or "invisible." I refuse to let the world dismiss me simply because they don't understand me or because I remind them of the fact that we only have so much control over our health. I don't want to be afraid to tell someone that I'm getting dizzy and need a break just because society says that I'm supposed to suffer in silence. I don't want to shy away from telling people what I'm feeling, or being honest with myself, because I'm afraid of judgement. Because, the truth is, I know a secret that society doesn't seem to know.

The truth is that my illnesses are a sign of strength, not a sign of weakness. As much as I'd love to return them, they have taught me resilience, healthy boundaries, empathy, compassion, and perseverance. They've turned me into an activist, advocate, and friend to many other disabled people across the globe. They have opened my eyes to the vast amounts of injustices in our world, and have given me a drive to fight them however I can.

Perhaps, most importantly, they have reminded me of

the inherent worth that each and every human being is born with. As a former over-achiever, I know how powerful the myth of 'good people work hard until they die' is. But, our value is not based on our ability to produce things or make money. The spoonies and disabled people who aren't activists, or advocates, or running the world have just as much value as those who are. Many of us try to hide our illnesses or disabilities away out of fear of judgement. Fear that those around us will think that we're weak or a burden. Fear that we'll be pushed aside and forgotten.

And that's why I share my stories with all of you. Why I rip open my scars and let you peek behind the bandages. I'm not going to be invisible anymore.

TALES OF A SPOONIE WARRIOR

Part One

WHO AM I, ANYWAY?

ANOTHER EXISTENTIAL CRISIS

'Who am I?' It's a question that seems to rattle through the minds of most of us, every now and then. Self-help books wouldn't be constantly flying off of the shelves if it wasn't for this desire that we all inherently have to understand ourselves and our place in the world. And I certainly am no exception.

In my late 20's, I found myself on one of these elusive journeys of self-discovery. It started with a 2,000 mile drive, a dissolving marriage, and an amazing group of people who helped me see myself clearly for the first time probably ever. I spent two grueling years working through anxieties, challenging my low self-image, and healing old wounds from the past. It was one of the most painful processes I've had to endure, yet it was completely worth it.

I spent most of my life, up to that point, in a cloud of darkness. Trauma I'd endured, starting at a very young age, only amplified every time I tried to bury it down. Once I started adding alcohol, drugs, and an eating disorder into the mix, trauma began to follow me around like a stray cat. Something horrible would happen, I'd try to bury it down or drink it away, which then led to something else horrible happening, so on and so forth.

Eventually, I went into treatment. I got sober and changed my life into exactly what I thought it was supposed to be. By 26, I had the husband, house, and child. The regular American Dream. But I was still suffering. My life was not my own. I was told to hide away parts of myself that I loved because they were thought of as unpleasant, or some other absurd descriptor. My then-husband and I went months without even looking at each other, let alone touching or exchanging kind words. I felt utterly alone, as I had my entire life, until I found myself.

Because of that journey of self-discovery, I learned to accept and love myself for who I was: loud, energetic, boisterous, friendly, optimistic, nerdy, goofy, talkative, and passionate about life. I accepted my old battle scars and found a way to break free from negative forces that had been feeding into my self-loathing. I began to see myself as worthy of love, and realized I didn't deserve all the abuse I'd been receiving for years, both from myself and others. I found a new zest for life, and a new desire to model all these qualities to my daughter.

I had been transformed! My daughter and I moved out of the house and found ourselves a new normal that we loved. I started reaching out to friends again, who I'd felt isolated from for so many years due to the cloud of unhappiness that followed me everywhere I went. I was exhilarated to work a job I loved, and even went on to find a new person (my current husband) who taught me what it means to be a partner. The future seemed wide open and full of possibilities. Life was now ours for the taking.

And then, once again, everything changed.

One day, I was bubbly, full of energy, and driven to work hard at the job I loved. And then, the very next day, while preparing for my students to perform a play I directed, I found myself shaking, weak, dizzy, short of breath, confused, nauseous, and drowning in fatigue. I was terrified. I had been fighting dizziness on and off for about six months before this, but I had assumed it was because I would push myself so hard, working around 60 hours a week, raising a child, completing a Master's degree, and being a dedicated yogi.

Going into the ER that day, I had no idea that it was going to be the start of a new life for me. Most of us think of illnesses as temporary. I'd hoped a shot or round of antibiotics would knock it right out. What I had not expected was for every single aspect of my newly formed life, the life I'd worked so hard for, to shatter.

Since that day, I've been diagnosed with Postural Orthostatic Tachycardia Syndrome (POTS) and Ehlers-Danlos syndrome – Hypermobility (HEDS). As it turns out, I had HEDS my entire life but had never been diagnosed. My symptoms had always been dismissed as something else, like growing pains or being naturally flexible. The major symptoms of POTS, however, were new to me. It hit me hard that December day of 2015 and has yet to back off. Even with medication and lifestyle changes, I still struggle every day to complete a fraction of what I used to be able to do.

At first, I denied that my diagnoses would affect my identity or life at all. I stubbornly held onto the hope that this would be temporary, simply a fleeting illness that would leave as suddenly as it appeared. Now, I know that it is most likely something I will live with for the rest of my life. That's the whole "chronic" part of "chronic illness" that I was refusing to acknowledge.

Honestly, I don't know if I can ever fully accept that this is forever. It's a hard concept to wrap your mind around. Maybe someday they will discover a cure? But, until then, I still have to learn how to live, and live fully, with my new disability. And so, I suddenly found myself thrown into the midst of yet another existential crisis.

Before POTS hit, I would dance and sing wherever I was; at the grocery store, at work, standing in line at Starbucks, walking up and down the stairs at home. My daughter and I would have dance parties daily where we would jam out to her favorite songs. I would sing her lullabies (well, if "Let it Go" counts as a lullaby) every night. I directed and acted in plays, something that I had been doing since I was a little kid. I would play games with my middle school students that had us running around the classroom together. I would go on adventures whenever possible and had a fairly active social life. It felt as though all of these things made me who I was, so where does that leave me now that I can't do any of them?

Even now, I still sometimes find myself feeling lost, confused, and angry. It often feels like I'd emerged from the storm only to be thrown right back in before I'd even finished drying off. There are days when I feel like I am falling, spinning, and reeling through space and I can't get my feet back on the ground. I lost a person I truly loved, myself, or at least the 'me' who I was back then, and I am not sure if I will ever find her again.

Now, I am tasked with the job of trying to find myself again. Well, maybe that's not entirely accurate. It's more like I am rebuilding myself. My illnesses tore down and destroyed so many of the building blocks that made me who I was before. I'm now searching for new building blocks as well as sifting through the wreckage to see which blocks may have survived.

I am still a mother, wife, teacher, daughter, sister, mentor, and artist. The way I fulfill these roles has changed greatly, but they are still part of who I am. I have not lost that. I cannot sing, dance, and act onstage, all things that I've spent my whole life doing, but I can write and maybe even find new ways to express myself. Due to the fatigue, I am not as energetic or boisterous as I used to be. However, I am still friendly, goofy, nerdy, passionate, and optimistic. I can't be as social as I want to be or as active in the world as I once was, but I am still here. I am still trying. And I still matter.

There are times when I will look back at what I used to be capable of and I end up feeling so small in comparison. Or I will watch others doing the things I wish I could be doing and feel jealous or sorry for myself. But I try to instead look at what things I do still have as well as what things I can still do. I get excited now by little accomplishments that I never would have thought twice about before, such as: sweeping the floors, a day without a headache, walking without assistance, surviving a social outing, a week without a doctor's visit, etc. I feel the 'old me' deep down inside screaming for the chance to dance, sing, and be the life of the party again. But then I think that maybe being able to do those things weren't as important to my identity as I thought they were.

Maybe I haven't really lost what made me 'me' after all. Maybe all of those actions and activities aren't as important as my attitude and spirit. Maybe in the mix of all of the things that I've lost, I have gained quite a few things as well. I'd like to think that through all of this I have become a little stronger, a little more understanding, a little more educated, a little more emphatic, and a little wiser. So, the challenge may not be in trying to find or redefine who I am. The real challenge is in finding how to hold onto who I am through it all.

MOBILITY & ME

I have two different mobility devices that I use regularly: a wheelchair and a rollator. A rollator is a lot like a walker, except it's on wheels so you don't have to lift it with each step and it has a little cushioned seat built in. My wheelchair is, well, it's a chair with wheels. My rollator is great for short trips, like going to the doctor's office or grabbing prescriptions, while my wheelchair helps me go places where a lot of walking would normally be required.

I love both Big Red (rollator) and Blue Steel (wheelchair) because they give me freedom to do things I otherwise couldn't. I am not bound to them, as most people say. I am liberated by them. And yet, I still have moments of weakness when I push myself too hard because I'm afraid of what judgement I might receive.

You see, there is a stigma around the use of assistive devices. For many abled people, getting a wheelchair, or walker, or cane, or rollator, is considered 'giving up.' It's seen as admitting defeat to your disability and deciding that this is who you are now. A popular line we're fed is "don't let your disability define you. It's all about mindset." Hmm. Even the perkiest of mindsets isn't going to allow me to climb up a flight of stairs, and while my disability may not define me, it's certainly *part* of my definition.

Here's what a lot of these "think it away" people don't realize: Whether I actually use my rollator or not, I'm still that same disabled person who needs one. The difference lies in whether or not disabled people will be shamed into suffering just to make someone else feel more comfortable in their incorrect beliefs. Because that's what they are asking us to do, to suffer for them. Well, I'm done with hurting myself to avoid judgement, and I highly recommend that any other disabled person who feels they need a mobility device to go ahead and get one.

However, I am going to issue a small warning:

If you are getting a wheelchair or a rollator, or really any kind of medical device, be prepared for odd looks, bizarre comments, and just general ableist nonsense. When I use my rollator to help me get around, whether it's the multi-storied building that houses my gastroenterologist's office or to a large restaurant, I get stares and whispers. "She's too young for that," someone sighs. "I bet it's her grandmothers," someone else clucks. But, don't let them stop you. You keep on rolling or strolling with pride.

There will also be people who make assumptions about you. For instance, I recently attended an event in my wheelchair. I was accompanied by some family friends who gave me a ride to the event and helped push me around. As we entered the building, we were greeted by a woman who kindly showed us some options for where we could park my chair. She then turned to my family friend and said, "she's so beautiful." It was dripping with the specific type of patronizing that is backed by a feeling of pride as the speaker believes they are showing how tolerant and loving they are while they're actually being very prejudiced. She then turned to me and slightly slower said, "You are so beautiful." "Uh, thanks," was all I managed to mutter out. Had we not been in the middle of a solemn event, perhaps I would have confronted her about her blatant ableism, but I decided to let it go.

So, yes. While in my chair or using my rollator, people have often talked slower or in a "child friendly" voice. There are others who stare at me with pity as I go about my day, not looking particularly pitiful, in my mind at least. There are many who won't look at me at all, unsure of how to handle seeing a disabled person out in the wild. They ignore me, look around me, or speak over my head, or simply talk to whoever is with me as if I have no authority over my own life.

There are people who roll their eyes, as if any 30-something with functioning legs who uses an assistive device is obviously just seeking attention. There's a litany of "what happened to you?" type questions and saintly looks given to my husband, because obviously he's a hero for staying with the likes of me. I mean, he kind of is, but it has nothing to do with my disabilities. I have received a wide variation of reactions to my use of assistive devices. The least common, but my absolute favorite, is when people treat me like a regular ol' human being like anyone else who just happens to need assistive devices.

I think it's important for anyone considering mobility aids to know that not everyone will understand your need for such a device, or even approve of you using it. Use it anyway.

I have heard many people in my various support groups lament over how they wish they could go to certain places or do certain things, but they don't want to use a necessary device because of the stigma or how people treat them while they're using it. It breaks my heart to hear it. Society already limits us in so many ways, judges us as lazy or fakers or as burdens; it is an extra dose of cruelty for them to then judge us for using devices that actually allow us to have some sort of independence.

I know this is easier said than done. I talk big, but I still feel hurt when I hear people laughing at my compression socks or giving me sideways glances for using a rollator. I cried when I had to give a graduation speech for my students from my wheelchair. I cringed as photos were taken of me while in my chair, angry that that was how I would be remembered. I have pushed myself too hard and too far because I was afraid of what people would think when they saw me with my chair or rollator.

These fears stem from the false notion that disabilities are shameful and should be hidden away. You shouldn't accept your disability as part of who you are, because disabilities are automatically considered negative, so claiming your disability is thought to be pessimistic and bad. It also comes from a fear of being thought of as weak, because we are told that disabilities are weaknesses.

Disabilities aren't shameful. Disabled people don't need to be hidden away or kept in the shadows. We shouldn't be made to feel embarrassed by our canes, walkers, wheelchairs, or rollators. They don't highlight our weaknesses, they add to our strengths.

My devices are so much more than mere equipment to me. They are my independence, freedom, and security. They are like old friends, welcoming me every time I turn to them, and supporting me through even the most difficult of challenges. They aren't fancy, or fashionable, but they are mine and I am incredibly grateful for all that they give to me.

Get whatever devices you need and use them proudly. Tell the naysayers to shove off, because you know the truth. Let your device be your secret weapon, rather than an anchor weighing you down.

DESCRIBING THE INDESCRIBABLE

Pain is a tricky thing, especially when it's chronic. It doesn't just dwell in one specific injured area. No, it spreads into your mind and soul, stealing your joy, hope, and sense of self. When the pain is at its strongest, it can feel as though nothing else exists except the pain and me. It's cruel, isolating, deceptive, and relentless.

Fortunately, my pain ebbs and flows, like the tide. It's always there, lurking, just some days it's more bearable than others. On lower pain days, I can do more. I can participate more in my life, go places, play with my daughter, bathe, or even have sex. On high pain days, all I can see is the pain. It wraps itself around my neck and slowly suffocates me.

It's so hard to explain exactly what this pain feels like, even as a writer. Sometimes, I have to leave the details to metaphors and verse, as they can capture the true essence far better than my clumsy paragraphs. Below is a poem I wrote trying to describe my pain as I was in the midst of a severe attack that left me bedridden and barely able to move for three months.

My Pain Is…

My pain is…
an uninvited guest
that overstays its welcome.
It greedily combs
through my life,
taking all I have to offer
and more.
Even when I think it's gone,
I find it has left crumbs behind
to remind me that
it's always with me.

My pain is…
a weighted shroud,
a suffocating film
that spreads across my body
devouring
every
inch.
It's crafted of broken glass,
jagged shards
woven together to create
a tapestry of nightmares.

My pain is…
an unforgiving fog.
It descends on me,
blocking out all light.
Hiding my thoughts
behind the cloud.
There they stay,
just out of reach,
waiting
for a momentary break
in the assault on my body.

My pain is...
a cold, twisting, metallic hand.
It wraps me in its embrace,
an ever-tightening grip,
and pulls me
down,
down,
down where I cease to be
and only the pain
survives.

My pain is a thief of all I used to be.
My pain is a whisper of lost dreams.

My pain is not all there is of me.

THERE GOES MY PURPOSE

I have started and re-started this part three or four times. I have written and rewritten drafts in my head and let my fingertips graze the keyboard, daring myself to start typing. I have been unsure of how to approach the topic of losing my career. Of how to do justice to the crushing feeling of loss that overwhelmed me as I came to the realization that I could no longer work and then said goodbye to the career I loved.

In attempting to express all I'm feeling, I had to ask myself: What really is the most important part of me losing my career? It's not listing off my resume or my education background. It's not explaining how I accidentally fell into teaching or even what subjects I taught. Actually, it's not really about teaching at all. No, to me, the most important part of this story is what happened to me once I became a teacher:

I found myself. I found my purpose.

That's right, as odd as it may sound, I found myself through my career. You remember that journey of discovery mentioned all those pages ago? Well, it started with my career. Actually, it started as I began the training process.

I was a Montessori secondary teacher. The training takes two summers and a few weekends in between. I remember, as I set off on the long drive to Texas, thinking that it was going to change everything. And it did.

I accidentally stumbled into teaching, yet I quickly discovered that, not only did I love it, I was actually pretty good at it, too. I was able to make learning fun, most of the time, at least. My passion, fire, spunk, empathy, creativity, and curiosity all were important tools to reach teenagers. And, watching them grow, learn, and discover helped me to grow, learn, and discover right along with them. It was hard not to feel like I was helping to make a difference in the world when I would watch my students bloom into responsible, caring, hard-working individuals.

Working with my students made me feel like I had a purpose in this life, as if maybe there was a reason for my existence after all. I'd spent most of my life feeling like I was a giant waste of space, so having a purpose to fulfill gave me a sense of belonging like I'd never felt before.

Letting go of that feeling of purpose is truly the hardest part of losing my career. Don't get me wrong, I still miss all the kids, field trips, games, breakthroughs, "ah-ha" moments, performances, laughter, smiles, and all of the other amazing things that existed in my classroom. But the most dizzying and disorienting part is feeling as though my purpose in life has been violently ripped from my grasp so soon after I had just discovered it. And if I don't have a purpose, then what am I doing here? What is the point of my existence?

The harsh reality is that they are just fine without me. They will be. Teachers come and teachers go. The school I worked at is a beautiful place and will continue to give kids a well-rounded education long after I was gone. I'm not the only person who could reach the kids and help them learn. The part that truly terrifies me is that I'm still unsure of how I will get on without them. Without that feeling of purpose.

Saying 'goodbye' to my job felt as though my entire world, everything I knew and had worked towards, was crashing down around my feet, but I'm the only one who can see it. I'm the only one who felt each and every earth quaking blast. There are others who felt the impact, for instance, my husband, Matt. His world has definitely been impacted and changed. But there are some changes that only I could feel. There are some changes that only I could see.

The suffocating panic over the belief that my only reason for existing in this universe was stripped away from me, was a feeling I carry alone. It was unsettling to watch everyone carry on about their day while I was in the midst of my world shattering. No matter how much I shared that feeling with people who cared, no matter how much I talked about it, and no matter how much they wish they could've taken the pain away, it was, and is, my burden to carry alone.

With my writing, I have attempted to find a new purpose. I hope that sharing my experiences and struggles will help others in their journeys. Because that's truly what I love the most, feeling like I've helped to make a difference in someone's life, feeling that because of something I've said or done, someone else feels a little less alone in the world. I always loved to write, so I threw myself into it, hoping that it would ground me as the chaos of change swirled violently around me.

Yet, I know the reality of uncertainty. I have watched as everything I've built up and created melted away within a matter of months. Living through so many major life changes has left me with an eerie awareness of the fragility of everything in life. I may not always be able to write. I've already met challenges with this as my wrists tire easily. So, if I continue to tie my purpose to actions and abilities, I am setting myself up to constantly fail.

It makes me wonder that maybe our purposes can change. Maybe it's not a fixed thing, but rather something that evolves and adapts as we grow. Maybe our purposes in life don't have to be tied to ability, production, or work. Maybe sometimes our purpose is just to be.

WHAT SOCIAL LIFE?

When Hurricane Harvey hit the southeast, we were left without power, water, and the internet for close to a week. This was hard for many reasons, including the fact that we lost an entire fridge and freezer's worth of food and had to endure the muggy gross hotness outside without an AC. But, it was the lack of internet access that struck me particularly hard.

Social media can have a very strong, very real, impact in the lives of people with chronic illnesses and/or disabilities. I've always been a very social person, but now I can rarely leave the house, which means that social media has become my main source of socialization each day. As I often tell my husband, "somedays it feels like my only access to the world outside of our home." That's a pretty powerful thing!

Now, I recognize that there are downsides of social media. The sense of anonymity often brings out the worst in many people. The comments sections read like toxic waste dumps. Bullying has reached new levels. People are unknowingly becoming famous due to videos or pictures taken without their consent that are used to mock or shame them.

Misunderstandings are common. You get the picture. However, the sense of participation that social media brings me is worth wading through all of that other crap.

When my symptoms are at their worst, I often won't leave the house for weeks at a time other than to go to the doctor's office. There is a whole world existing out there and I want to be part of it, even if I can't leave my bedroom. Social media allows me to do that.

There are a bunch of people with chronic illnesses and disabilities on social media. Not long after I was diagnosed with POTS, I found support groups online. Since that day, I have joined several different groups, and have become an active member in various communities on FB, Twitter, Instagram, and Pinterest. These groups and communities can really only be found online. I'm sure there are local support groups for disabilities and chronic illnesses in many cities, but as many chronic illnesses make getting out of the house to socialize difficult, well...you can understand why it can be difficult to attend regularly.

Through social media, I have been able to find a place among my peers. I have learned so much about my own illnesses, as well as many others. For many people it's a distraction or frivolous extra. For me, it can be a lifeline.

When I'm in a bad flare, or struggling with depression and anxiety, I know that I can turn to these communities for understanding and support. Even with an extremely supportive spouse, it is an amazing feeling to be able to connect with people who just "get" it. Without ever having met any of these people in person, I feel tied to them as we share both the highs and extremely low lows of our illnesses. My online friends can help lift me up in laughter as we crack jokes about our common experiences, or cry with me as we mourn our losses together. While it doesn't take the pain away, it makes it a little easier to handle.

There are many disabled and chronically ill people out there who don't have supportive spouses, family, or friends. There are many who live with people who refuse to accept the reality of their illnesses, and even deny them access to care. For them, these online communities are the only source of caring and empathy they see. When access to doctors is limited, learning how others with the same illnesses treat their symptoms can save them a lot of hurt and pain. Even just having someone say, "I believe you" is a powerful thing that many people don't get outside of these groups. The value of having your experience validated by others cannot be overstated.

And yet, it is a concept that seems to escape many who haven't had to experience it themselves. I have seen multiple people say crap like, "if you can be on social media, then you can work." These people don't seem to understand a) how different being active on social media is from having a full time job, or b) how important the ability to connect with other people is for everyone. There seems to be a widely held belief that if you can spend time online then you can work, and that if you can afford internet and/or a phone then you don't need government assistance of any kind (including disability). It's a toxic line of thinking used to deny people basic human rights because they haven't "earned" it. (That sound you just heard was of me scoffing)

People complain about Welfare recipients, or any kind of government assistance, using funds to pay for internet services or spending time on social media instead of working 24/7 at finding a job. It is absurd to think that someone should be denied this sense of community just because they aren't wealthy. Without access to social media, I would never have sought the advice of Dysautonomia experts at Vanderbilt, or pushed my doctors to screen me for Ehlers-Danlos syndrome. I would never have discovered many of the treatments I use to help me cope with my illnesses. I wouldn't have found my voice as an activist. My life would look incredibly different today without access to social media and these communities.

For so many, social media is just a fun activity, but for some of us, it's the key to the whole world.

EARNING WARRIOR STATUS

Fight. Be a fighter. This expression is used a lot in our culture. We talk about fighting for rights, fighting for your dream, fighting institutions, and, even, fighting illnesses. While the same word is used, the action itself looks very different in each of its uses. Hell, it even looks different from person to person.

I call myself a Spoonie Warrior, so obviously I believe that I'm fighting in some way. There are some who don't think I am because of their bias around what that battle looks like. People who think that calling myself disabled, leaving my job, getting mobility devices, and even taking medications are signs of me giving up. These people are wrong.

For some illnesses and diseases, it's easy to see how someone is fighting. Mind you, I am not saying that the fight *itself* is easier, it's just more clear-cut how the fighting is done. There's a diagnosis and a cure. The cure is the tool of the fight. It could be a surgery or a medicine or something similar. But the fight has a clear beginning, middle, and end.

For other illnesses and diseases, such as the ones I am lucky enough to have, the fight isn't so clear cut. It's messy, it's non-linear, and it's poorly defined. Even if there is a cure, it isn't always cut and dry. Sometimes it's like a roll of the dice and you never know if you'll be the winner or not.

As mentioned above, my illnesses don't have cures. EDS, POTS, PTSD, and the multiple other letter groupings I deal with can only be managed, not removed. There are some people who help fight these illnesses by funding research in hopes of finding a cure. They do fundraisers and raise awareness to try and call attention to the impact these illnesses have.

That's an important way of fighting, and I take part when I can, but it's only a very small part of my reality. The truth is, my body is waging a war on itself every single day. It would be impossible to explain every single way I fight, so I'm not going to try. Instead, here are the top weapons in my arsenal used to battle my illnesses:

1. Medication

Lots and lots of medication. You would probably be surprised how many medications I have to take on a daily basis just to be able to function somewhat well. Our medicine cabinet at home looks like we're trying to start our own pharmacy, or stockpiling for the zombie apocalypse. But, each medicine does something specific that the others don't do. They work together like a well-oiled machine. Removing one proves to be detrimental to my well-being.

But there's another side of the medication fight. There's an inner and outer struggle over how many medications I take. There's a guilt that comes with being medicated. Believe me, if I could go all natural, I would. If I could heal myself with just my diet, I would. While diet can help ease some of my symptoms, unfortunately, eating a handful of cashews a day is not enough to fight my PTSD and get me off anti-depressants. No amount of kale or leafy greens will keep my heart rate and blood pressure in check. And I have tried eating an apple a day, but it just doesn't seem to keep the doctor away.

The guilt that comes with requiring an entire pharmacy to keep you functioning comes from the latest trend of medicine shaming. It seems like every day a brand new meme goes viral telling those of us that use medicines that our medicines are only making us sicker, making us require more medicines, and that if we would only eat such and such root then all our problems will be solved. I can't tell you how many times I have had a discussion with a person who knows nothing about my illness but feels that they know enough to tell me that my doctors are poisoning me, Big Pharma has brainwashed me, and that all illnesses are figments of our imagination.

Or worse, they implicate that I'm the reason that I'm still sick because I'm too lazy to try their miracle cure. Just as our culture likes to victim blame, they like to patient blame as well. According to memes, posts, rants, and conversations I've had with various people, I wouldn't be disabled if I just tried harder, exercised more, ate the right foods, prayed more, went to the *right* church, and really truly wanted to feel better. Having to face the reality of being chronically ill is crushing enough without being told that it's all your fault for being that way.

Now, I'm not knocking natural medicines, or eating healthy, or prayer, or whatever helps you. Trust me, I don't like spending a small fortune each month at the pharmacy. What I am knocking is the ableist idea of medicine shaming, and the attitude that people with chronic illnesses are too lazy to get better. We have enough to deal with, without arguing with narrow-minded people who believe their 30-second conversation with us makes them qualified to question our treatment. Spoiler alert: it doesn't.

2. Doctors

I go to so many different doctors. I have a primary

care physician, who basically just serves as a referral vehicle since there isn't much that she is able to treat herself. I have a cardiologist/electrophysiologist, rheumatologist, neurologist, psychologist, psychiatrist, gastroenterologist, and a physical therapist. I wish that there could be just one doctor who I could see to treat all of my illnesses, but that is not how medicine is practiced. My illnesses affect every system, therefore I see a specialist for each system to help keep them all in check.

Each new doctor brings with it their own obstacles. I have to fight with insurance to get them to cover it, because why should a 30-something year old woman have to see so many specialists? Then I have the anxiety of meeting the new doctor. Will they understand my illnesses? If they don't understand them, will they be willing to research them and learn more? Or will they be one of the many doctors that dismisses my illnesses as being all in my head since they have never heard of them?

Finding supportive doctors is a must when you have a rare (or rarely understood) illness. They are an incredibly important weapon to have. However, there are also some not-so-understanding medical professionals out there. They become a fight all of their own. Even just trying to decide whether or not to go to the ER is a battle since I often end up leaving feeling worse than I came in thanks to the stress and anxiety the ill-informed doctors and nurses put on me. I've had nurses insinuate that I'm a hypochondriac because I come in using the actual medical terms for my maladies, assuming I must have looked up the names on WebMD instead of being given the names in a diagnosis. But what other choice do I have? To just pray whatever symptom I'm fighting isn't going to kill me? Rock, meet hard place.

I'm not trying to insult anyone in the medical profession. I have great respect for people who dedicate their lives to saving the lives of others. But the stigma against people with invisible illnesses and/or disabilities often bleeds into the medical field as well. I have to fight to be taken seriously, as many professionals dismiss any symptoms they don't understand as being "anxiety." Anxiety is a serious issue, but it has become a kind of catch-all diagnosis for illnesses that aren't well understood, which leads to poor treatment.

The fact that my illnesses aren't well understood can also lead to doctors or nurses with good intentions giving me the wrong treatment. I was hospitalized for bradycardia last summer and while I was there, the doctor stopped the nurses from giving me one of my regular medications. They didn't believe I needed it. They also fed me a "cardiac friendly" diet, which means very little salt. I'm on a special diet that requires a lot of salt. I mean, A LOT! No matter how much I insisted, since they weren't able to reach my regular cardiologist, they refused to alter the diet. I left the hospital that weekend feeling much worse than I did when I got there.

Fighting to be heard, and believed, by people in the medical field was not something I expected to encounter, but it has become a major part of my regular life.

3. Being Active

Well, really I mean being as active as possible whenever it's possible, but "being active" just sounds better as a section header.

Being active for me now, looks very different than what I would have called being active before becoming disabled. Before December of 2015, I was highly active. I was notorious for taking on too much work, then working myself ragged to get it all done. I was full of energy. I danced and sang wherever I was, no matter who was looking. I bounced around, often literally, from activity to activity. Radiating energy was kinda my thing.

Now, I get dizzy from walking down the drive to get the mail. In fact, as I write this, I'm trying to calm my racing heart and I feel a headache coming on because I had to mop up a water spill on the floor. I can no longer bounce from activity to activity, I can no longer bounce period. I can't remember the last time I danced, a realization that immediately has tears prickling behind my eyelids.

When compared to how active I used to be, I don't seem very active at all, actually. But that's why I try really hard not to compare my old self with my new self. As soon as I do, I start to spiral into an aching sadness, a mourning of who I used to be and all that I'd hoped to become. So, let's not talk about that right now. *sniff sniff* We've already been down that road and don't need to go back.

There was a period of time, after I first got POTS, when I wouldn't do much of anything at all. I was afraid of draining all of my resources. But now, I try to use my limited reserve of energy (or spoons in chronic illness speak) in ways that are worth it. Because, honestly, some things are worth the flare.

Picking up my daughter to comfort her when she's hurt is worth the dizziness I feel later. Spending time with friends and family on special occasions is worth the day or two, or week, of rest I need after. Even writing leaves me dizzy and fatigued, but it gives me much more than it takes away. I mean, what's the point of having spoons at all if I can't use them when I need them?

However, there are also days when I want nothing more than to be with my daughter playing, but I can't get out of bed. When I want to see my friends or family, but the fatigue is too overwhelming. When I want to go to the activity or event we planned well in advance, but the pain is too strong. There are days when I listen to Harper and Matt playing and laughing in the living room and I would give anything to be where they are, to be laughing and playing along.

My illnesses don't care how much I want to be who I was before. They don't care how infuriating it is to feel like I'm missing out on so much of my daughter's childhood. They don't care how many weeks I have to take off from writing, or how many novels have been left unfinished. They certainly don't care how many plans I have to cancel, no matter how much I was looking forward to them. They don't care, because they are illnesses. They exist in me whether I want them there or not and no amount of wishing or positive thinking will change that.

So, I fight for those moments when I can be there, no matter how few and far between they may be. I fight to create new ways to be with Harper, to just be present with her whenever I can. I fight to give all that I can, even if it's only a small fraction of what I used to be able to give. And I fight to accept my new limits, no matter how hard that is to do.

4. Talking

Anyone who knows me, knows that I've never had an issue with talking. However, since becoming disabled, I've changed the way I talk and what I talk about. The thing I talk about most is, you guessed it, my illnesses.

I talk about my illnesses because they are a huge part of my life. They impact pretty much everything I do. As I've said before, they may not define who I am, but they certainly are part of my definition, so staying silent about them feels like I'm being dishonest about who I am.

I also talk about them to normalize it. I don't think that chronic illnesses are something dirty or shameful, yet they are often treated that way. It's seen as taboo to talk about them or shine light on them. Or the person doing the talking is thought to just be seeking attention or sympathy. I've dealt with that last assumption a lot. I assure you, I am not seeking attention and I loathe pity. If someone reacts to me telling my story with those feelings, it says a lot more about their biases than my intentions.

I share my struggles because I know that I'm not the only one going through this. I'm not the only one who feels this way. I'm not the only one who struggles the way I struggle. I speak up for those who can't, or aren't ready, to speak up for themselves. There are so many reasons why I refuse to stay silent about my experiences, but we'll explore that more later.

5. Love

It may sound cheesy, but I think there's something to

that whole "love is all you need" thing. I mean, clearly it isn't *all* I need, we've already covered the whole doctors and medicine thing, but it is certainly an important part of my needs. My illnesses have shown me just how strong and powerful love truly is.

On the worst of the worst of my days, the love I get from my husband, my daughter, our family, and my friends keep me going. On days when I can't find the strength to fight, they fight for me. My partner in life, Matt, researches my illnesses, spends hours scouring the internet for recipes I can actually eat, drives me to and from every one of my doctor's appointments, and never ceases to amaze me with how understanding he can be.

Why does he do this? According to him, it's because he loves me and would never even think for a second to do any different. And he's not the only one. I have been overwhelmed by the kindness that I have been shown by so many people that I love. Whether it's my dad texting every day to see how I'm feeling, my best friend sending me funny pictures to make me laugh, Harper trying to "help" push my wheelchair, my former students mailing me a get well soon card, a friend driving over to bring me dinner, my mother-in-law playing detective in the grocery store to find things that I can eat so that I don't feel sick after dinner, or the countless other amazing and wonderful things that the wonderful people in my life have done to show how much they love and care about me.

Having chronic illnesses can also show you what relationships you might need to let go. When family and people you thought were friends start preaching about how your illnesses are your fault, or all in your head, or you're just milking it for attention…that's when you realize that maybe these people don't have your best interests at heart. And when you are running on limited stores of energy, you don't have any to spare for toxic relationships. Let that shit go and let more love in.

My love for others helps me to fight as well. My love

for my daughter, Harper, helps shake me out of my worst days. It helps to warm my heart when I'm in the depths of my sadness. She helps me to be stronger, because I want to show her what strength looks like. My love for Matt helps me to work past my anxieties, to process trauma that I've kept hidden for a long time, and to be more forgiving of myself.

Trials in life can often make people angry and bitter. Believe me, I definitely have my moments when I am angry. I get angry at the universe for making me this way, angry at the world for not understanding, and angry at myself for not being better. It's the love of others, and my love for them, that keeps that anger from rising up and taking over. This love is the only thing that makes it possible for me to fight in all those other ways that I've mentioned. It reminds me of what is good in this world, of what is worth fighting for.

It is love that makes me stronger. It gives me hope even on the darkest of my days. It shows me that I am so much more than my ability to dance through the halls or sing at the top of my lungs. And, it helps me to remember that no matter how insignificant I may feel, I still matter to some, and that means the world to me.

A WALKING CONTRADICTION

Hey guys, guess what? I have anxiety. Yup, a whole bunch of it. I know, you're probably thinking "there's no way she has *real* anxiety. She's too loud, boisterous, and completely extroverted." Well, you're not wrong. I am all of those things, but I am also a chaotic mass of anxiety thanks to years of abuse bringing on PTSD.

In the last few years, anxiety seems to have become more accepted and normalized...but only a certain manifestation of it. You see, there's still a stereotype out there that attempts to put all people with Anxiety Disorders in one small box: those with anxiety are all shy, quiet, reserved, and introverted. Yet, I am living proof that that's not always true.

I have always been a friendly, talkative, outgoing person. I grew up on the stage and never met a stranger. And yet, I have an anxiety disorder. Most of the time when I tell people this, they can't believe it because I seem too confident and gregarious to have anxiety. Whelp, ladies and gents, that's why stereotypes suck. People often stop seeing each individual person and only see the artificial box they've created.

In the efforts to smash stigmas and break free of stereotypes, I'm sharing with all of you how my anxiety manifests itself differently than expected. If the following relates to you, then you might be an extrovert with anxiety, as well:

1. You talk too much

There are a lot of people with anxiety who have a hard time speaking in front of crowds, talking to new people, being on the phone...basically anything around talking to people who aren't in a small inner circle. For me, it's far easier to talk to strangers than people I know kinda well. I can go up on stage and play any character, never missing a beat, but ask me to speak as myself and I'm riddled with anxiety. The worst part is that the more nervous I get, the more I talk. I accidentally overshare way more often than I'd like to admit, mainly because my anxiety kicks in and I start babbling about whatever comes to mind.

This has led people to believe that I'm wildly confident, open about all my flaws, and fearless of judgement. Ha! The truth is I'm anxious and terrified the entire time, but I just can't stop myself from talking. And the more I talk, the more anxious I get as I recognize that I'm rambling on and oversharing, which only leads to me rambling and oversharing even more. I have spent many a night cursing myself for something horrifying I said when anxious, even years and years after the original conversation took place.

Even sharing as much about myself as I do in my writing sometimes feels more like an impulse than a choice. I spend hours reeling in anxiety every time I publish a new post. The only thing that keeps me going is the fact that I believe the benefits outweigh the risk. Or, maybe I'm just a glutton for punishment? At least when I'm writing, I can edit and revise my words to avoid complete verbal diarrhea. Unfortunately, that's not an option in daily conversations.

So, people who told me my entire life "you talk too much," I would have to say I agree. But sometimes, I just can't stop myself.

2. You have "resting nice face"

You've heard of "Resting Bitch Face?" Well, I have the opposite problem, "Resting Nice Face." That means that my natural look is one that screams, "Come talk to me! I want to be your friend and hear all of your stories!" It can be a struggle to get people to take me seriously, and I have to work twice as hard as regular-faced people to let others know that I'm angry. Plus, as friendly as I am, sometimes I don't want everyone in the grocery store stopping to tell me about their daughter's divorce, sister's surgery, and postal worker's acne.

Part of "Resting Nice Face" is that I smile at people all the time. I wish I could say that I'm every smile is because I'm always happy and confident or that I'm just trying to bring cheer to everyone I meet, but that's not always the case. Sometimes I smile because I think I might know you and I'm anxious that if I don't smile you'll think that I'm a horrible human being and run off to tell everyone just how much of a monster I am until everyone hates me. Sometimes I smile because I was zoned out when you suddenly glanced at me and smiling is the first thing I can think of to make you think that I'm not a creeper or in the midst of a breakdown. Sometimes I smile because I'm scared and I truly hope that, if I smile, you'll like me and therefore be less likely to hurt me. Yep, anxiety takes you from 0-60 pretty damn fast.

This is another habit of mine that has tricked people into thinking I am confident and sure of myself. Little do they realize how much anxiety drives it. It has also led to the uncomfortable situations mentioned above, where strangers are taken in by my welcoming attitude and will share things that I am not prepared to hear, but I'm too anxious to tell them to stop or to walk away so I just sit there, smiling, while waiting for the conversation to end or death to come.

3. FOMO and FOGO

"FOMO," aka "Fear of Missing Out," is another

strange dilemma in outgoing people with anxiety where two opposing ideas wrestle for attention, as FOMO meets FOGO (my newly coined term for "Fear of Going Out.") Before going out and socializing, particularly with people I don't know or don't know well, I'm riddled with the anxiety of what might be. I play over possible conversations in my head, plan out for worst-case scenarios, and rehearse important things ahead of time like pronouncing names correctly or remembering how we met. Once at the social event, I am consumed with the anxiety that everyone is going to discover what an awkward mess I truly am. Did I laugh enough at that joke? Or did I laugh too much? I don't know what that word means, did they notice that I don't know what it means?? Will they see how much I'm sweating?! These questions, and more, race through my mind for most of the event and lead to the over-talking, oversharing, and over-smiling mentioned above.

And yet, as much as I stress about going to, and getting through, an event, I'm filled with a whole different kind of anxiety around not going. I start to worry that someone will be mad that I didn't show up, that I've let people down, that people will realize they're better off without me, that my friends will stop inviting me places, or that something amazing will happen and I'll miss it. I mean, what if it turned out to be the best night of my life? How can I not go?? I struggle to leave an event, especially if I'm having fun, because I worry that I'll end up regretting it.

I get this little recognized type of anxiety I like to call the "carpe diem anxiety." It's where I frantically worry that I am not seizing each day enough, that I'm not savoring each breath like I'm supposed to, that life is going by fast and maybe I haven't done enough with it. I spiral into stressing about how there are things I've done that I'll never be able to experience in the same way again, and what if I didn't enjoy them enough the first time around? Am I just forever ruined? Is my life just passing me by, or am I really living it?? Existential crisis are common place for me.

4. You're a social chameleon

For my entire life, I've had the ability to fit in, at least partially, with most groups I socialized with. While this is sometimes a good thing, it can also come at the expense of me ignoring my own personal or moral boundaries. If I'm in a group and someone brings up an idea or says something that I don't agree with, my anxiety kicks in. I worry about what will happen if I tell them 'no,' or walk away, or disagree? I become terrified that they won't like me, that they'll hate me even, and I become anxious of what might happen if they do. That includes letting people treat me poorly, make fun of me, and take advantage of me. I've been part of multiple "friend" groups where I was basically the punching bag for cruel jokes, but my anxiety around being alone or being hated led me to put up with it for far longer than I should have.

To an outsider, I looked like a vivacious social butterfly who gets along with everybody, but they couldn't see how few genuine connections I had because I would only let most people see the bits of myself that they found agreeable. Very few people saw the whole me. I use past tense here because this is one problem that I have made great improvements on in the past few years. Maintaining healthy boundaries and asserting my needs is still difficult, but I continue to get better at it each and every day.

Now, you may find yourself saying, "Why is she complaining? A type of anxiety where you appear confident? I'll take it!" There are definitely some benefits of this type of anxiety, but there are also a lot of downsides. The most important downside being that it is much harder to get people to take your anxiety seriously. For a long time, I didn't even recognize these symptoms as being anxiety related, because they looked so different from what I was told most anxious people looked like.

Just as there is no one way to be disabled, there is no

one way to have an Anxiety Disorder. Most of my anxiety stems from my PTSD and the abuse I've endured, which has left me with inappropriate 'life or death' feelings around people liking me or, at least, being happy. Anxiety comes from multiple sources and shows itself in many different ways. Don't discount someone else's experience just because it doesn't look the way you think it should. Bottom line: you have no idea what someone else is living through, so start listening more than judging.

SAIDEE WYNN

Part Two

MAKE 'EM LAUGH

WHAT THE HELL IS A SPOONIE?

My self-appointed title of "Spoonie Warrior" has inspired many questions: "Am I a spoonie," "what *is* a spoonie," and "where do you get off calling yourself a warrior?" Skipping the last one, let's talk about spoonies. In short, a spoonie is a nickname for people with chronic illnesses. It was inspired by an article called "The Spoon Theory" by Christine Miserandino. The basic gist of it is that "spoons" represent energy. People with chronic illnesses often have a very limited number of spoons, while healthier individuals have a much larger amount. Spoonies have to assess how many spoons each activity in life will require, as we only have so many to dish out. Most non-spoonies don't have to consider how many spoons a shower will cost, and if it will leave enough spoons to actually get dressed after.

So, if you have a chronic illness, no matter the severity of it, you are a spoonie. That's the quick and easy way to know if you're a spoonie. But where's the fun in that?? Using my own personal experiences, and those of other spoonies I know, I've compiled a list here of signs that you may be a spoonie, served up ala a famous '90's "Redneck" who was a fan of lists.

Now, don't anyone go spoiling the fun by claiming I've diagnosed them with a chronic illness through this list. I'm not a doctor and know nothing about you (yes, you, the one reading this now). Really, this is just my creative way of detailing, and laughing about, the common spoonie experience.

I present you with "10 Signs You Might Be a Spoonie:"

1. If You're the Youngest Person in the Waiting Room…

Apparently, many of my specialists seem to mainly cater to older clientele. I suppose it's because, other than the chronically ill, most younger people have far fewer health issues requiring less visits. At most every visit, I am the youngest person in the waiting room by at least 20 years. The other patrons will sneak quizzical glances my way, probably trying to decide if I'm actually a patient, or just someone's driver.

It's not always a bad thing. I tend to relate the most with older patients because we often have the same symptoms. At family gatherings, my husband's grandmother and I often end up sharing stories of our medical experiences, a lot of which are the same. The other day I was making a long trek into the radiology wing of the hospital. I had my rollator and passed about three different senior citizens using walkers, all of whom joked with me about the difficulty of the trek and how much it sucks. Having the joints and gastro system of a 60 year old means I relate better to them than most people my age, health wise at least.

If you ever, at any point in your life, have experienced frequently being the youngest patient at your doctor's office, then you might be a spoonie.

2. If your wish list is full of medical devices & accessories…

Birthday coming up? Get a new wheelchair padded seat. Christmas? A brand new blood pressure cuff. Hanukkah? Eight pairs of compression socks. Arbor Day? Some new

Kinesio tape will do the trick. My current wish list is filled with medical devices, device accessories, and clothing that helps to raise awareness. Just this past Christmas I received Kinesio tape, rollator decorations, a wheelchair bag, and an exercise ball…I couldn't have been happier.

Medical devices and accessories add up fast and most often aren't covered by insurance. I've spent hundreds of dollars on compression wear alone! That's what makes these items such great gifts. We get something that helps alleviate symptoms, and the giver gets the joy of seeing us squeal in delight as we finally open up the new water bottle we'd been eyeing for months.

If you ask for spoonie gear for gifts for any occasion, then you might be a spoonie.

3. If you have favorite hospital staff in the emergency room…

I try so hard to stay out of the Emergency Room (ER), I really do. Yet, due to the nature of my chronic illnesses, I still end up going there at least once every few months. Matt and I joke that they need to start a ticket punching system for spoonies, where every 10th visit is free. Needless to say, my frequent visits have allowed me to get to know the staff fairly well.

I've had doctors choose to treat me instead of letting another doctor take me on when I'm in the ER, because they remember me and remember my conditions. I've had nurses that recognize me when they see me rolling in. I certainly don't know them all, and they don't all know me, but you know you're a frequent flyer in the ER when there is any amount of recognition at all.

Therefore, if you spend enough time in the ER that you have favorite staff members, you might be a spoonie.

4. If your medical records could fill their own cabinet…

As of the end of April 2017, a year after my initial application for disability, their file on me was 998 pages in length. Since then, I've had countless doctor's visits, medical tests, procedures, and ER visits. My disability file only includes medical records from the past year and a half, since that was when I became disabled by my conditions. And that's only counting since I became disabled. I had many doctor's visits, tests, procedures, and treatments before POTS thanks to the high injury rate of EDS. I feel pretty confident that, in all, my medical records put together would easily fill an entire file cabinet of their own.

Being chronically ill tends to come along with lots and lots of medical records, so, if your records could fill their own cabinet, you might be a spoonie.

5. If you know more about your condition than most doctors…

Once I found out that I had Ehlers-Danlos syndrome (EDS), I realized that most of the doctors that I had sought answers from for years were taking shots in the dark, and that none of the answers I had been given ever came close to explaining what was going on with my body. This taught me that I had to learn to be my own advocate and work as hard as I could to understand my conditions better. This has led to me often knowing way more about my condition than most medical professionals I talk to. I spend a ridiculous amount of time researching my conditions as well as any possible treatments for them.

When you have a rare, or rarely recognized, illness, you have no choice but to learn all about your condition. Getting treatment from a professional who doesn't understand your specific needs and symptoms can lead to major health problems. That's why most of the spoonies I know are some of the best researchers I've ever met. We trade medical journals the way others swap recipes. If there's a new treatment option or medical discovery for a chronic illness, chances are spoonies will be among the first to find out.

If you know more about your condition than most medical professionals who you meet, and do enough research to be a second year medical student, then you might be a spoonie.

6. If you have enough supplies to start your own pharmacy...

Between the medications, supplements, OTC remedies, medical devices, and other random products, our house somewhat resembles a slightly less organized drug store. Our supply seems to be growing daily as I encounter new symptoms and need new remedies to help with them. If I were to suddenly be cured, I'm pretty sure we could survive for at least a few months by functioning as a small pharmacy or convenience store.

If your home resembles any type of pharmacy, you might be a spoonie.

7. If a hospital bracelet is your idea of expensive jewelry...

According to the intake nurse at the hospital I frequent, the average ER trip is around $2,000. That's more than I have ever spent on any piece of jewelry in my entire life. It seems like you're charged a minimum of $500 just for walking in the door, making those little plastic bracelets they send you home with worth a pretty penny. While I wouldn't mind having a beautiful gemstone ring instead of these tacky bangles, they are unfortunately a necessary part of having chronic illnesses.

I almost feel bad tossing them in the trash knowing how much I'll be paying for them later. They come in a few subtle variations, which is always fun, but they are mostly the same. Thick, plastic, and near impossible to rip off.

If these plastic bracelets are among the most expensive jewelry you own, you might be a spoonie.

8. If you have a "good" vein...

I have one good vein, just one. If my blood pooling is bad, then the veins in my hands also stick out, however, they tend to roll or the IV will pull since my skin is so stretchy.

Therefore, I always direct nurses to the one good prominent vein in my right arm. That means that this vein is often abused.

If I have multiple visits in one week requiring IVs and/or blood draws, I end up with a very tender and bruised arm. At least knowing which vein is my good vein typically saves me from the pain of multiple sticks, unless I get too dehydrated, that is.

If you tend to point out your good vein to nurses, you might be a spoonie.

9. If you constantly get unsolicited medical advice…

Honestly, I have so much to say on this that I could write an entire chapter on it. Instead, you're getting an essay that you can find later on in this book. In short, it's a common spoonie experience that none of us enjoy.

Common unsolicited medical advice include, but are not limited to: "You're too young to have those issues," "but you don't look sick," "it's all in your head, you just need to relax more," "my friend's sister's cousin took a semester of chiropractor school and says your illness is completely curable with vitamins," "essential oils will fix it all," "if you just <insert random advice on diet, supplements, shamans, prayer, positive thinking, and/or exercise here> then you'll be cured." There are many many more, but these tend to be among the most popular.

If everyone seems to have an opinion on your illness and how to cure it, you might be a spoonie.

10. If you see your doctor and/or pharmacist more than your friends…

I am at the pharmacy at least once a week, thanks to different medicines being refilled at different times. The longest period of time I go between visits with a specialist is 6 months. If I'm having a particular issue, then I may end up seeing them every week to every two weeks. I also seem to have at least two stretches a year where I have at least one doctor's appointment a week with various different doctors for a good month or two.

With it being so difficult for me to get out of the house often, I have friends I haven't seen in years even though they live nearby. Even with my closest friends, I only see them about once or twice a year. It's easy to see how my social calendar is mostly filled with medical professionals, leaving a lot less room for family and friends.

Yes, if you see your doctors more often than you see your friends, you might be a spoonie.

This is in no way an extensive list of the common experiences of those of us with chronic illnesses. I could've gone on about a love affair with dry shampoo, the hatred of pressure changes, the necessity of streaming services, and more. But, I've gotta have something to write about in my next book, so I'll stop with these.

MY FAVORITE CLEANING HACKS

Even before I became disabled, cleaning wasn't exactly my favorite pastime. Floors often went neglected, windows were left grimy, and dishes piled up in the sink. Still, it was fairly easy to keep the house an acceptable level of clean by putting in a quick 20 minutes of cleaning a night. Oh boy, those were the days!

Thanks to my Postural Orthostatic Tachycardia Syndrome (POTS), and the exercise intolerance it brings with it, 20 minutes of light cleaning leaves me gasping for breath, flushed in my face, dizzy, drenched in sweat, and with a racing heart. With three humans and two pets, mess accumulates quickly in this house. It's as though each living creature in our home travels with their own personal sized cyclone that leaves wreckage wherever anyone goes.

Needless to say, we've had to get creative with how we pick up around the house. Please be advised that these tips may not work for everyone...so don't get mad at me if your house is still messy after reading this piece. If nothing else, at least these brilliant (untested) hacks can leave you in a brighter mood while you stare at the disaster that is your home.

1. Put Your Feet To Work!

Many of us spoonies spend the majority of our days in bed or restricted to the couch, only getting up to go to the bathroom or to the kitchen for more supplies. Spending half an hour or more walking around the house, up and down stairs, and into every room is too much activity for many of us, so why not break the job into smaller chunks? Simply wear a pair of super fuzzy socks and you'll be cleaning wherever you go! You can even sweep from the couch by simply gliding your feet around the floor without ever getting up. Once the dirt has all been lifted, soak them in hot water and soap and you've got travel size mops ready to go. Sure, most of the cleaning might be constrained to the path from the couch to the kitchen and bathroom, but ya gotta start somewhere! Now, this may not work if your floors aren't visible under mounds of stuff...but, then again, if ya can't see it, then how do ya know it's even dirty?!

2. Save Water, Clean Your Body & Your Clothes

Most spoonies know that bathing isn't exactly easy. Personally, I have to rest for at least 30 minutes to an hour after bathing just to get enough energy to get dressed. Using so many of my daily allotted spoons on bathing doesn't leave much for cleaning or other chores. That's what makes this idea so brilliant! You can cut down on your chore time by washing your clothes as you wash your body. You're already lathering up, why not spread that lather around and get everything clean at once? Besides, washing clothes one outfit at a time also saves on folding...although it won't do much for the laundry pile that is growing in the hall. But, that's why we call these life "hacks" and not life "solvers."

3. Invest in Pets

Pets are great for many, many reasons. They provide companionship, entertainment, and joy. And, yes, they do create some messes of their own, but they will also make sure that you never have to clean up spilled drinks or dropped food ever again! It's true, while not highly advertised, pets love to help clean up messes.

In fact, our animals are so dedicated to their jobs as

cleaners that they immediately come running anytime a package is opened that they believe might possibly have even a morsel of food in it. They will then faithfully watch our every move, our every bite, just to make sure that should any food hit the ground they will be able to clean it up right away. They'll even go so far as to sniff the area for hours after we've finished eating, just to ensure that they've fully completed the task.

I don't even want to think about the great number of crumbs that would be filling our home if it weren't for our hardworking faithful companions. Not to mention the time they could save us on washing dishes, as they are more than willing to lick each and every dish until it is spotless! [Warning: If you don't have a fenced in yard to let your dog go outside without you having to walk them, then you may end up wasting all the spoons you saved on dishes on walking the dog. Non-shedding breeds are recommended. Proceed with caution.]

4. Decorate Creatively

You know what they say, "it's all in how you decorate." Do they say that? Well, I'm sure someone says that. Think outside the box and soon your mess will turn into dazzling designs. For instance, a colorful shawl draped over a dresser can hide the mail that has piled up on top. A vase of fresh cut flowers can mask the smell from the overflowing trashcan. Stack empty pizza or shipping boxes to create a unique end table or footstool. Used containers from Chinese take-out are great decorative additions for any table top and can be filled with all sorts of goodies found around the house, such as: batteries, loose change, rubber bands, paper clips, that one sock without a pair, and so on. A bright and cheerful blanket transforms any laundry pile into a pure work of art. Guests are sure to be left wondering where on Earth you learned to decorate when they see your creative style.

5. Just Apply Philosophy

If all else fails, I like to get philosophical with my cleaning habits. Many a philosopher has pondered, "if a tree falls in the woods and there's no one there to hear it, did it make a sound?" I simply apply that way of thinking to the room around me, "if no one can see the mess, is it really there?"

There are many ways in which this can manifest itself in a spoonie's life. For starters, keeping the lights dimmed works wonders. Bright light has a way of showing off all the dust that has collected around a room, but if you keep the lights down, then no one can see the dust and it's almost as if it isn't there at all. Keep your blinds down on all of your windows, that way you'll never have to see the smudges. And, in extreme cases, simply forbid people from ever entering your home. No one will see how messy it is if they aren't allowed inside!

In all seriousness, please don't take any of these suggestions seriously. Or, if you do, please remember to record it and share the video with me so I can get in some good laughs.

Keeping your house clean while also trying to stay alive is hard, and I don't know that any of us have a magic fix worked out (if you do, please let me know). We're all trying to do the best we can with what we've got, and for that, I think we're pretty freaking awesome.

WHEN A SPOONIE EXERCISES

Exercise is important. We all know that, we've heard it many times. It helps with circulation, muscle tone, and sends lovely endorphins coursing through your body. It helps keep your blood pressure, blood sugar, and cholesterol levels in check. Plus, it gives you an excuse to wear your favorite yoga pants and sport a messy bun (which I do constantly anyway). It's also used as a favorite bit of unsolicited advice given by abled people to explain why us disabled and/or chronically ill people are still disabled/chronically ill.

Being able to exercise is a privilege. You probably didn't realize that, especially since so many people dread exercising and have to talk themselves into doing it. That's why gyms start gimmicks such as giving out free pizza at the door just to try to get people in. However, just because someone isn't exercising in the way you think they should or to the extent that you think they should, does not automatically indicate laziness or a lack of desire. Not everyone's bodies are capable of withstanding exercises.

There are many of us out there who have what's called exercise intolerance, where our bodies essentially freak out if they try even simple exercises. Luckily, one of my medications helps me with my exercise intolerance and allows me to do some small simple strengthening activities, but it is slow going. At times, I've been able to work up to 20 whole minutes of exercise a day! To a non-spoonie, that doesn't seem like much at all. For me, it's like I'm climbing freaking Everest every single time. It is difficult, it is exhausting, and I face many, many setbacks, but building muscle is the only thing that will keep my joints in place.

What better way to teach people about the struggles of exercise intolerance, along with EDS and POTS, than by sharing my innermost thoughts that I have every time I attempt to get moving? Hopefully, it also helps some fellow spoonies recognize that they are not alone in their struggles. Or, it can just help us all to blow off steam with some good ol' fashioned belly laughs.

3:00 pm- "I should probably do my exercises so that I have time to recover before dinner." *stares blankly at the closet where my exercise equipment is held*

3:15 pm- "Ok, I definitely should start exercising now. Here goes nothing." *I put on a bra, a dreaded task, and slowly rise up out of bed. I carefully peel each electrode pad from my tens unit off of my body and place them tenderly on their plastic protectors. After a quick trip to the restroom, since standing up makes me have to pee due to a stretchy bladder, I'm ready to go.*

3:20 pm- *I pull my extra-large yoga mat out of my closet and unroll it on my floor. Already my heart rate is climbing.* "Surely this counts towards my exercises."

I proceed to begin exercises given to me by a physical therapist:
--**hip stretches**-- "shoulders back, am I winging? Shit, I'm hyper-extending. Engage the core, re-position my rib cage, there's that winging again...oh crap, tuck in my chin, no swan necks. Ok, stretch....dammit, hyper-extending again!"
--**back twist**-- "how far should I twist? How far is normal? Oops, was that a good pop or a bad pop? Ugh, hyper-

extending again, engage your damn core."

--**hip raises**-- "which muscles am I supposed to be working here? My thighs? That feels interesting. My back? Nope, that hurts. My stomach? That seems right...oh crap, I went too far again. Pull in your belly button, engage your core."

--**arm & leg extensions**-- "Ok, engage the core, don't hyper-extend your back...good, wait, what is that clicking sound...why is my hip clicking?" *moves leg in different directions until clicking stops* "ah, ok, so that's how hips are meant to move...crap, forgot to engage the core again. Oh man, I don't even know what my shoulders are doing right now. How do normal people move their arms?? Dammit, ENGAGE YOUR CORE!"

--**plank**-- "Where are my shoulders supposed to go? Are they winging? I can't feel if they are winging! I need a spotter just for my shoulder blades. Crap, engage your core, your butt is dropping. Shit, tuck in your chin, no swan necks."

--**child pose**-- "ah, this feels nice. Why can't all exercises feel like this? Surely this is building up some kind of muscle."

--**standing to roll up the mat**-- "ok, remember to rise up slowly...." *sits back down until spots leave the field of vision* "ok, let's try that again...slowly" *rolls up the mat while trying not to pass out as room spins around me and my heart rate increases*

--**recumbent bike**-- "Start slow, don't push too hard. Easy going...why does my hip keep popping?" *quick adjustment* "That's better. Crap, stop freaking hyper-extending your back! ENGAGE YOUR DAMN CORE!!! God, my head hurts...there's that swan neck again...I don't even care what my shoulders are doing anymore...are my eyes shaking? Can eyes shake? Why do they feel like they're shaking? Ok, don't just stop abruptly, cool down...I think I'm cool enough."

3:40 pm- "Let's check my heart rate. 170? Ok, maybe the bike was a bad idea. How long was I on it...5 minutes?!?! Ugh! I need water, and salt, and my heating pad, and my tens, and sleep." *I lay back on my bed, allowing my heart rate to calm

down to its normal rate. The room is spinning and my eyes still feel like they are shaking. I am hot and cold at the same time.*
As I slip back into my comfort zone, I quietly whisper to myself, "engage your damn core."

Now, not all spoonies will experience the same things as they exercise. Since I have Ehlers-Danlos syndrome, part of my battle is trying to figure out how to move my joints without hyper-extending them, the other part is trying not to pass out thanks to POTS. That 15 minutes of exercise uses up about half of my spoons for the day.

All of that is to say: if you ever feel the need to tell someone that they aren't trying hard enough to get better, please remember, the things that may come easily to you (such as standing up without passing out) do not always come easily to others. For my fellow spoonies out there, whether you can exercise 5 minutes a day, an hour, or not at all, you are a warrior and you are rocking it. And, remember, it's ok to laugh at yourself once in a while. Oh, and engage your core.

Part Three

SOAP BOX

NO, IT'S NOT ALL IN MY HEAD

There aren't many places in our society where a person feels as incredibly vulnerable as we do at a doctor's office. We trust doctors with our lives, in every sense of the phrase, which puts doctors in a very unique position. We have no choice but to trust them, as we don't have the extensive knowledge of the human body, understanding of medications, or ability to perform complex medical procedures the way doctors can. There are many doctors who understand the true depth of that trust and respect it. However, there are many doctors who seem to have forgotten what their responsibility to the patient is, or, even, that they have a responsibility at all.

Not too long ago, I ended up in the ER with a heart rate of 40bpm, severe lethargy, and shortness of breath. As I've said before, I try really hard to stay out of the ER, because it's rare to find a doctor who understands my condition, but I knew that there was a possibility of this being life-threatening. When explaining to the doctor about how all this started within an hour of trying a new medicine, he laughed at me and said, "Well, just stop taking the medicine," and then shook his head as if I had just asked if buffalos have wings.

There I lay in front of him: the heart monitor blaring because my heart rate kept setting off the alarms, barely able to keep my eyes open because of the overwhelming fatigue, and shaking from the chills. And, yet, he felt that it was appropriate to make me feel as if I had wasted his time by coming into the ER to receive care.

That evening something in me clicked and I decided that I would not sit through another horrible visit where nothing is accomplished and I end up with a bill for $2000. I tried to be patient and calm, but I didn't have enough spoons to do so. I turned to the doctor and asserted, "Could you please just go ahead and let me know if you're actually going to take me seriously and treat me, or not, today? Because I don't want to waste my time or money if you're just going to laugh at me and pretend that nothing is going on."

He began to retort with the familiar, "You seem a bit hysterical," but I cut him off declaring, "Don't even start the whole 'you're upset so it must just be anxiety crap.' Yes, I am upset, I'm upset because you don't seem to be taking me seriously, not because I have anxiety."

I'm not quite sure where that bravado came from, but I'm glad that I said it. After that, the doctor apologized to me multiple times. He even spoke to me as if I was a peer instead of treating me like a six-year-old child (as many doctors tend to do). He treated me like a human being with a right to understand my illnesses, which, unfortunately, is not a common way to be treated by doctors. I am often greeted with disdain when I ask multiple questions in attempts to understand what is going on in my body, as if I should accept it as enough that they have come up with a description for my symptoms and any further information is unnecessary.

Now, not all doctors are like this. I've had a few wonderful doctors who are willing to sit and talk to me for however long is needed so that I can better understand the ins and outs of my illnesses and symptoms. I have doctors who are willing to admit when they don't have the answers and either promise to research to learn more or help me find a doctor that does understand. I've watched as a doctor turns to their computer to search my illnesses right there in front of me, which shows me a willingness to learn and understand that I appreciate greatly. There isn't any shame in medical professionals admitting that they don't have the answer; there is shame, however, in them trying to convince a patient that they are making up their symptoms in order to cover up the fact that the doctor doesn't understand their illness.

In the many online support groups that I participate in, one of the most common complaints is having doctors who don't believe us when we say what we are feeling. It's hard for someone without a chronic illness to understand how disheartening a "normal" test result can be when you are desperate for an answer as to why you are feeling the symptoms you feel. The crushing disappointment isn't because we want to be sick, rather, it's because we already know that we *are* sick. We need a test to confirm it not only to be able to start a treatment plan, but to also show our doctors that our symptoms are real. We desperately want to be believed.

One reason that this is such a common occurrence for people with chronic illnesses, is that a lot of our symptoms are self-reported. Pain, for instance, is completely subjective. There is no way for a doctor to strap you to a machine to measure how much pain you are feeling and where the pain is coming from. The only way they know is through what the patient is telling them. Even seeing a broken bone on an x-ray doesn't tell a doctor what level of pain their patient is experiencing.

There are many symptoms that don't show up on tests. Nausea, headaches, migraines (for the most part), muscle pain, joint pain, fatigue, chest pressure, on and on…you get the picture. Tests can sometimes help show the cause of these symptoms, but they can't measure the effect that each of these symptoms have on the patient nor the intensity that each patient feels. For some doctors, that means that if they can't find a reason for your symptoms, they believe you must be making them up.

Growing up with undiagnosed Ehlers-Danlos syndrome, I was no stranger to this kind of disbelief. People, my doctor included, often wouldn't believe that I could really be injured as often as I said I was. And surely I couldn't really be sick as often as I said I was. I was often accused of attention-seeking and hysterics, which led to me keeping my symptoms a secret unless they reached a level of pain I could no longer ignore.

This kind of disbelief leads to constantly second-guessing yourself. I still do it to this day. If I have certain symptoms and tests keep coming back "normal" then I start to question myself, wondering if it really is all just in my head. I will try to will it away or ignore it in hopes that if I don't believe in it myself, then it can't be real. This method has yet to yield any positive results.

Around a year ago, I was bedridden for several months from excruciating pain. It stemmed from my left hip all the way down my left leg. It caused horrible nerve pain that extended into my pelvic region and caused severe issues with using the bathroom. My gastroenterologist ran all the tests she could think of until ruling out a gastrointestinal problem. She then said that it could be a pinched nerve and that my next step would be to see a neurologist.

My first visit with the neurologist was scary, but promising. She seemed to take my symptoms seriously. She said that I had definite neuropathy in my left foot and believed there was some kind of issue stemming from my lower back. She sent me for an MRI to confirm. That's when things went downhill.

When I came back in after my MRI, she said that it was perfect. In fact, she said she'd never seen such a healthy spine MRI. I was frustrated, of course, because I was still in horrible pain and wasn't any closer to figuring out what was wrong with me. I didn't expect, however, for her treatment of me to change so suddenly.

She looked at me with accusing eyes and said, "Why are you in the wheelchair?" I reminded her that I have POTS, which makes me dizzy upon standing, and that I was still in severe pain despite what the MRI showed. She asked me to get up and walk down the hall. As I slowly made my way, she asked, "Why are you walking like that? You're walking like you're afraid to walk." I, again, reminded her of both my POTS and severe pain. She told me that she would refer me for a nerve study but that she was pretty sure it was going to come back normal and that she couldn't see anything wrong with me. She then began to question my use of different pain medications, medications prescribed to me by a different doctor, as if I was drug seeking. I explained the painful nature of EDS and reminded her that I hadn't asked her for any prescriptions.

I left angry, frustrated, and still in pain with no idea where to go next. I went into a deep depression, wondering if her implications were right and that it really was all in my head. Then, a friend reached out to me and said that my symptoms sounded very similar to a condition called Piriformis Syndrome. Obviously, she couldn't diagnose me, but she hoped that it could help point me in the right direction.

I did what I always do when there is a chance for an answer and dove into research. I began to treat myself as if I had Piriformis Syndrome, as I was desperate and sure that it wouldn't hurt if it turned out to be something else. I attacked the problem aggressively with my home TENS unit, heating pad, stretches, and medications I was already prescribed. Slowly, but surely, I started to see amazing results. I still fight with it to this day, but it has improved exponentially. I spent months crying most of the days away because of how severe the pain was. Now, it's become a minor inconvenience.

There are multiple reasons why this kind of attitude from doctors is harmful. But, to me, the absolute worst part is how it makes us question and doubt ourselves. We leave these doctors feeling broken, beaten down, confused, lost, and hopeless. And, thanks to insurance, we don't always have anywhere else to turn. If one doctor decides that you aren't really sick, they can cause all possible treatments to come to a halt.

Now, I know that there are people out there who have a mental illness that causes them to make themselves sick or to make themselves look sick. I know that this is a real thing. Anxiety is also a real issue that can manifest itself in multiple different ways, as I discussed earlier. But, that is one of the many troubling aspects about this "it's all in your head" phenomenon. It is most often used as a way to dismiss a patient and their concerns, rather than out of concern for another mental health condition. If a patient has anxiety so severe that they are unable to get out of bed due to the pain, telling that patient to "stop worrying so much" isn't just dismissive, it's neglect.

We've all heard of the Hippocratic Oath, the oath all doctors take where they swear, among other things, to "first, do no harm." For a doctor who is refusing to treat a patient because they don't believe their symptoms are real, how are they not causing great harm? I now have anxiety before meeting any new doctor, simply because of how often my very real symptoms have been dismissed. How can the doctors who dismissed me claim that they haven't harmed me? I went 30 years without being diagnosed with EDS, doing unknown amounts of damage to my joints, because my doctor didn't believe me. He absolutely did harm.

Trust is a precious thing. In most cases, it has to be earned. Doctors get, and expect, our trust as soon as we walk in the door. And yet, many do not act in ways that are deserving of that trust. Sure, they may be great for a broken bone or cancer, things that can be clearly seen and defined on tests, but they are letting down the chronic illness community. For those of us with mysterious illnesses that are rarely understood, we are denied that same level of belief and caring, while being asked for the same level of trust and respect.

After 30-some odd years with my body, I know it pretty well. While a doctor who has just met me may be able to name all the bones in my hand, they haven't felt the pain I feel with too much movement, the clicking when I wave, or the popping that happens when bearing weight. For doctors to properly treat chronic illnesses, they need to start believing their patients. They need to start listening to our concerns and search for answers, instead of dismissing us. No, I'm not saying that as soon as a patient shouts "I have pain" then doctors need to throw strong pain medicines at them or whatnot. But they need to recognize us as partners in our own treatment plans rather than outsiders.

To any doctors who may be reading this: Please, believe us when we say something is wrong. We may not know what the problem is or why it is happening, but we know our own bodies better than anyone else does, so we know when something is off. We are coming to you for help, not to waste your time. We are scared, frustrated, and confused. We are seeking understanding and comfort, not judgement and dismissal. If a patient has attempted to self-diagnose, try to understand why they have done that. It's most likely because they were desperate for answers that they weren't getting anywhere else. Most importantly, remember that your patients are people, not just medical charts.

SO OVER IT

While I'm relatively new to being disabled, I've technically had chronic illnesses my entire life. Even before being diagnosed, my illnesses affected my life greatly, I just didn't realize that they were the ones causing the trouble. Most people will want to hear that, despite any difficulties, I make sure that I live every day to the fullest and I always find the silver lining in every gray cloud. Well, just because most people want to hear that, doesn't make it true.

The truth is that I get tired. I'm not just talking about "need to take a nap" tired or even the full body aching of constant fatigue. No, this kind of tired is a general feeling of "I'M SO OVER IT" that is typically accompanied by a desire to shed myself of my illnesses and every bit of misery they bring with them. By reading posts from other spoonies in various support groups and such, I have come to learn that I'm not the only one who feels this way. So, based on those interactions and my own personal feelings, I now bring to you Eight Things Spoonies Are Totally Over:

1. Invalidation

I'm gonna go out on a limb here and say that *everyone* wants to be validated. We want to know that our beliefs and experiences are recognized as true and valid by others. It seems to be a very natural part of the human condition.

For people with chronic illnesses, we want our pain and symptoms to be validated. We want to be believed. As I've mentioned multiple times, in the 30 years that I lived with an undiagnosed chronic illness, I had frequent injuries and was often sick. Every new injury came with people who would deny my pain. "There's no way you can hurt yourself that often," "you just want attention," "you're so dramatic," "it's all in your head," "just get over it." As I type out those phrases that I have heard a countless number of times, my throat begins to tighten up and my heart rate increases because these words kept me up at night for years. Believe me, after 30-something years of being invalidated, **I am over it**.

This goes beyond physical pain and illnesses. As an abuse survivor with PTSD, my mental health symptoms are also often dismissed and ignored as well. One might even argue that this invalidation is even more common for mental illnesses, when posts about medicine shaming and "nature cures depression" going viral daily. Either way, it manifests itself quite similarly. Belittling phrases get tossed around, just as with physical illnesses. Phrases like: "Just exercise more," "do yoga," "stop being so negative," and "just think happy thoughts." None of them are helpful. All of them are harmful.

No matter if your symptoms are physical or mental, this kind of invalidation is powerful. It seeps into your pores and affects how you see the world around you. You start to doubt your own sense of reality and learn not to share these parts of yourself with others. You try to hide away your pain and sadness. You try to swallow those parts of you deep down and lock them away. However, pretending your illnesses don't exist won't make your illnesses go away. Believe me, I've tried. And someone else pretending that my illnesses and/or symptoms don't exist won't make them go away either; it will only teach me that you are someone who I can't trust to be myself with.

2. Misrepresentation

Representation is important. Disabled people are not

often represented in our media & entertainment. When disabled characters are present in media & entertainment, we are typically misrepresented. Most movies, books, TV shows, etc., that actually show disabled characters center around a main theme of a person overcoming their disability, choosing to risk their life or take their life because of their disability, or how altruistic the people who love those with disabilities are (because we're obviously all burdens to others). These stories are most often written, directed, produced, and acted by abled people. So, no matter how hard they try to be accurate, they will always be approaching our disabilities from an abled point of view.

Another popular theme is that of people faking their disabilities. We've all seen the memes depicting a person who stands up out of a wheelchair with an accompanying snarky comment about "a miracle in the alcohol aisle" or something equally ill-informed. Memes such as these reinforce the false notion that people who can walk just use wheelchairs because they are lazy or attention seeking or whatever. As a part-time wheelchair user, I have been afraid to use the electric chairs at stores because I'm afraid I will end up on a meme talking about how lazy I am. Especially after a man was almost beaten to death when walking away from his car in a handicap parking spot because someone believed this abled trope that all disabled people must be permanent wheelchair users.

Misrepresentation is harmful. It harms all of us. It harms me when I see it because I am reminded that society expects me to prove my disability to them. It harms disabled people with invisible illnesses when strangers harass them for using a handicap parking spot or a motorized scooter at the store simply because they don't "look" disabled. It harms visibly disabled people when society tells them their life isn't worth living. It harms society when we refuse to acknowledge and validate the existence of so many disabled people. And, you know what, we're over it.

3. Pain, Pain, and More Pain

Now, not everyone with chronic illness necessarily has chronic pain, but mental pain can be just as debilitating as physical pain. The whole chronic part of our illnesses means that they are ongoing. They are the equivalent of the Energizer Bunny of illnesses. Some people get periods of relief between the moments of pain. Some people have various levels of pain, but are always in pain of one kind or another. No matter how often the pain attacks happen or how long they last, we are over them.

For as long as I can remember, I seemed to bounce from one injury to another. I would also get bugs, viruses, and infections back to back. As soon as one illness or injury would begin to heal, another would swoop in to take its place. I once had strep throat 4 times in one year. This has only been magnified since becoming disabled by my illnesses. Every time I think I've got a handle on my symptoms, some new issue comes bubbling up to the surface to rock my world all over again.

As mentioned above, this often leads people to not believe me when I say that I've injured myself or caught some virus. The other effect it can have is that people become tired hearing about my pains. I mean, shouldn't I be over it by now? I *am* over it. I am *so* over it. Unfortunately, that doesn't stop my body from hurting. If you are tired of hearing me complain about my illnesses, imagine how tired I must be of living with them.

4. Missing Out

Recently, my daughter came home with a picture she drew of our family while she was at school. The picture showed her, Matt, and our dog all playing outside the house. Where was Mommy in the picture? I was a floating face smiling down on them from a window in the house. That picture crushed me. Even as I write about it, I start crying all over again.

I do a lot to try and stay present in my daughter's life. I

push myself to use up every spoon in my reserve on days when I know I can, just so that I can soak in every moment of her childhood possible. But, I miss out. I miss out on a lot. I don't get to take her to parties or play dates. I don't get to run, dance, or sing with her. There are many things that I want to do with her that I just can't.

I miss out with my friends as well. I have friends who live within 20 minutes of me that I haven't seen in well over a year because I'm often too tired or in too much pain. I make and break friend dates frequently because my condition changes on a day to day, sometimes minute to minute, basis. I want to go on adventurous vacations. I want to have lunch dates with my friends that last for hours because we can't stop talking. I want to be in a play, or take a class, or even just enjoy a hike through nature. Believe me, when people with chronic illness cancel plans or flake out, it's not because we don't want to see you, it's because our bodies won't let us. And, you guessed it, we're over it.

5. Exploitation

The other day I was approached by someone online who was attempting to sell me some miracle cure or whatever, and you know what, I was honestly just about desperate enough to do it. I normally don't buy into these pitches, especially from people I don't know, but I was in a bad place and was tempted to try anything. Something the guy said sent red flags flying up for me, so I started to ask him some questions. Pretty quickly his story began to unravel and he began pushing harder and harder for me to buy some of his miracle elixir. He said to me, "I wouldn't take advantage of a disabled girl." Except, yes he would. As will thousands of other people.

My openness about my illnesses has left me wide open for these kinds of exploitation. I have had people pitch just about every kind of juice, powder, oil, exercise, and supplement out there. I've read articles that boast to have found a cure to my ailments only to find absolutely zero evidence to support its efficacy. I get messages nearly daily from people who are eager to take what little money I have, and I am so over it.

I am over people looking at me and seeing money signs instead of a person. I am over people trying to take advantage of the fact that I am hurting so they can line their pockets. Chronically ill people are vulnerable to these kinds of attacks not because we're not intelligent, but because many of us are so desperate to feel better. And yet, when we don't try out the latest health craze on the market, we are branded as being too lazy to try to get better. Believe it or not, our illnesses do not exist merely for your monetary gain.

6. Waiting

We are always waiting. We're waiting for a doctor's appointment, test results, medicine to kick in, medicine to wear off, pain to subside, the next flare, the flare to end, research, and cures. We also wait for people to understand us, to listen to us, to believe us, and to support us. The waiting goes on and on, in a seemingly endless stream. And, surprise, we're over it.

Waiting for pain relief is one of the hardest things to wait for, but many of us do it every single day. I have days were I wait for pain relief and nothing I try works. I may find a medicine that seems to be help, but in less than two weeks, the pain comes back. Then I am thrown right back into the waiting, again. Waiting for more relief, waiting for the doctors to take my pain seriously, and waiting for something to finally work. On top of all of this, I am still waiting to get approved for disability benefits so that I can stop worrying about money every second of every day. I'm so tired of waiting. I'm ready for results.

7. Isolation

Chronic illnesses are isolating. They just are. No matter how many supportive friends and family members you may have, there will always be some feeling of isolation. There are parts of your illness that you can't share with others, no matter how understanding they are. I like to believe that I'm a fairly talented wordsmith, but I still lack the ability to fully explain the weight of my pain, fatigue, sadness, and loss.

I spend most of my time in my house. Lately, a good portion of my time at home has been spent in bed. If I leave the house, it is usually to go to the doctor. Occasionally, I'm able to get out to see friends or family. My ability to leave the house is especially hindered by the heat of summer, which only adds to the feeling of isolation. The world keeps on spinning outside my window, but I only get glimpses and snippets of it through pictures and stories from others. I wish that I could break through the shroud of isolation, but I have yet to find a way. And, yes, I am over it.

8. Fighting

Yes, I'm a fighter. I fight every single day of my life. I'm proud of my determination, but I'm also so over having to fight in the first place.

I've been praised for my strength and bravery in the face of adversity, but to me it doesn't feel like something worth praising. See, I don't feel like I've ever had a choice in the matter. To me, to live means to fight. Even when I lay around in bed all day, I am fighting against pain or fighting to get some sleep. To exist is to struggle, that is the life I have known.

And I am tired of it. I'm exhausted from the constant fighting. I don't mean that to sound like I am tired of living or existing. I just wish it were possible to clock out of the fight. I would love to be able to take a vacation from my illnesses, to be able to go even just a day without having to think about medicines, salt, fluids, compression, pain, or spoons. But my body doesn't work that way. I don't get that option. So, even though I am so tired of fighting, I still fight.

Chronic illnesses come with so many unexpected symptoms, and these eight are just a handful of them. The hardest part is that no matter how over all these things we are, we know they won't disappear overnight. Asking nicely has yet to end invalidation, exploitation, misrepresentation, or any of the many issues we face. But, maybe if we keep talking about it and shouting it from the rooftops, then maybe things will eventually shift. Until then, I'm so over it.

BUT, HAVE YOU TRIED YOGA?

There's this odd medical phenomenon that surrounds people with chronic illnesses. It seems, few doctors can treat us, zero doctors know how to cure us, and yet, every layman who has ever tried yoga or juicing seems to believe they have all the answers to our ailments. They can't pronounce our diagnosis, but they watched a life-changing documentary so now they know the true secrets of the universe.

Look, I get it. They see someone hurting and want to help. Maybe they were sick once but because they tried x-supplement or y-exercise they now feel better, and that's great. I'm happy for them, really, I am. And I appreciate the sentiment of wanting to help others to feel better. I understand that most of these people genuinely are trying to help. That's why I think it's important for anyone with these habits to understand why it's not helpful and actually ends up hurting us instead. That's how I came up with this list of "Five Reasons Unsolicited Advice Hurts More Than It Helps:"

1. I know my illnesses better than most doctors
As I've mentioned multiple times, spoonies are avid researchers. I wouldn't have even gotten the diagnoses that I have if it wasn't for me researching and pushing to be evaluated. When POTS first hit, I took to the internet to learn as much as I could. That research led me to Ehlers-Danlos

syndrome, something I'd never heard of before, yet every single thing I read about it was like reading a detailed account of my life. That's what led to me asking to be screened and, inevitably, being diagnosed with EDS, with several other doctors confirming the diagnosis.

On TV, doctors try tirelessly to find out what is wrong with their patient and get them the proper treatment. Unfortunately, that isn't usually reality. That is what makes researching such a necessity for us. Most everyone I know with a rare chronic illness has done enough research to earn an honorary MD. Anytime there is even a hint of a treatment that helps, we are all over it like ants at a picnic, researching all possible effects and benefits. The chances of a random non-medical professional person knowing more than me about the intricacies of my illnesses are incredibly slim, unless they actually have my illnesses.

Perhaps this advice wouldn't be as frustrating if the person giving it took the time to talk to me about my illnesses and symptoms, and seemed genuinely interested in what I'm going through. Yet, that's not usually the case. Most of the time this "curative" advice is used to stop any conversations about my illnesses or symptoms. It's as if by telling me to go on a juice cleanse, that person has demonstrated that they care when they really don't, but now they feel they can move on in good conscience.

Or, they can move forward with the assurance that if I don't get magically better, it's my fault so they don't have to care about it anymore. When someone tells me, "If you just stop letting those doctors poison you, you'd get better," what I hear is, "if you tried harder then you wouldn't be sick, so obviously you're not trying hard enough and I refuse to enable your laziness by showing any empathy." Ok, maybe the word count doesn't quite match up, but that's the general subtext spoonies are hearing.

2. 'Natural' doesn't necessarily mean safe

I'm all for natural medications and treatments

whenever possible. Diet can help with the severity of some of my symptoms, talk therapy and EMDR treatments help my PTSD more than any of my pills, and building strong muscles can help with my joint pain. I'm also a huge advocate for federally legalized medical marijuana (MMJ) and CBD oil, as it has the possibility to help a huge amount of people. I, personally, could get off of at least half of my medications if I was able to use medical marijuana. It has far less side effects than most of my medicines and has the benefit of being all-natural. Honestly, I don't understand how it's even still up for debate.

However, that doesn't mean that every treatment labeled 'all-natural' is beneficial for all people, or anyone at all. Sometimes these treatments are merely placebos. Even for treatments that do benefit some, it won't necessarily benefit everyone. Not only is every illness different, but every patient is different as well. Caffeine in espresso beans is all natural, but it still gives me horrible tachycardia. I know spoonies who've had bad reactions to MMJ. Turmeric is a good natural anti-inflammatory, but I still can't take it due to erosion of my stomach lining. There are many things that will cause us a lot more harm if we try it, especially since so many of us have unusual allergies or sensitivities. So, we research (see above), or wait until scientists have been able to research the effects of a treatment on patients like us. Until we have that evidence, it's not always worth it to try.

Even more importantly, just because something is all-natural doesn't mean it's safe, especially when being self-administered and the dosage is random. I've had people tell me, "It's all-natural so you can take as much of it as you want because it won't hurt you," and that is some incredibly bad advice. Arsenic and Cyanide are natural. Belladonna is used in very small doses as a muscle relaxant, but is incredibly fatal if using the incorrect dosage, which is why it was given the nickname of "deadly nightshade." Many natural things are poisonous or toxic to humans in either small or large doses. We can't just go running into the woods eating every berry, mushroom, and herb we come in contact with if we want to survive to leave the woods, so why are so many people so willing to pretend that all-natural means 100% safe?

I know the popular belief is that traditional doctors want us to stay sick because they benefit off of us being ill, but practitioners of holistic medicine also benefit off of us being sick and needing repeated treatment. Correct me if I'm wrong, but it's typically not free to go to any kind of holistic practice and they typically don't take insurance either, so it's all out-of-pocket. If they could cure everyone they saw within a few visits, they would surely be out of business in no time. Just like with medication and treatments, someone saying they're all-natural doesn't mean they are effective or safe. Snake oil salesmen exist in all types of medicine.

3. We don't like medicine...we NEED it

The general consensus among my fellow spoonies is that we hate being on a bunch of meds, spending a fortune at the pharmacy, and dealing with an array of side effects. We don't take the medicine because we enjoy those things, we take it because we need it to be able to function. If a medicine is not helping us, generally that means we stop taking it. We tend to not just sit around throwing a bunch of useless meds down our gullets for the heck of it.

The judgement tends to get especially harsh when it comes to pain medicine. There are definitely people who abuse pain medicines, but more often than not, they are buying those meds in the grocery store parking lot or some shady location rather than actually receiving a legitimate prescription for them. There are many patients out there who need access to pain medication regularly who are not using it to get high, or to abuse it, but are using it for an actual medical need; yet the stigma and war on pain medication has made it far more difficult for us to have access to these medicines. This, to me at least, extends to the crusade against legalizing medical marijuana, as it is an incredibly effective chronic pain medicine with far less side effects than narcotics and opioids.

I know I've already talked about medicine and the stigma towards those of us who rely on them, but that's because it is a pretty big deal. When a well-meaning person tells me about how all my medicines are peddled to me by greedy doctors to keep me sick and that I should just try yoga/oils/vitamins/juicing/fasting/whatever else instead, it hurts me. It fills me with guilt about the medicines I have to take. It's even gotten me to try to go without my medications, with disastrous results. It's pretty clear to me that this is an incredibly dangerous stigma.

4. We don't enjoy being ill

The worst effect of these types of "helpful" conversations is that they typically end up with us feeling anxious, guilty, and angry; while the person giving the advice ends up feeling either relieved from having done such a good deed or convinced that we just want to be sick. I have had someone tell me that I'm just too negative and not willing to get any better. This is perhaps the worst thing you can say to someone with chronic illness or illnesses.

In case I haven't already made this clear enough, IT IS NOT OUR FAULT THAT WE ARE SICK. It's not because we have too much negative energy, or didn't pray enough, or prayed to the wrong god, or any of the other various things that people claim have made us ill. When people imply, or even flat-out tell us, that the only reason we are still sick is because we aren't trying hard enough, it crushes us. The guilt and hurt are suffocating as we try to imagine in what world would we willingly put ourselves through so much pain, so many tests, and losing so much of our previous lives. That's like telling someone who just watched as every single one of their valued possessions burned up in a fire right in front of them, that they really wanted it to happen.

5. Health often comes down to luck

My husband is pretty healthy. Other than some dental problems, his systems all run fairly well. I've actually only seen him sick once in the past three years. Other than cutting his finger, he never really has injuries. What's his trick? Genetics. In spite of eating a diet of half good healthy foods and half gas station junk food, as well as never exercising and maintaining some bad habits, he has yet to be suddenly stricken bed-ridden, like I am.

When I was knocked down by POTS, I was the healthiest I had ever been. I was eating a mostly vegan & mostly whole-food diet, doing intense yoga daily, taking very few medications, drinking tons of water, and staying very active both at home and work. By all accounts, I should've been invulnerable against illnesses of all kinds. I was doing all the "right" things, after all. And yet, I still got sick due to a genetic condition I was born with.

Our habits can certainly have an impact on our health. Exercise can make it less likely to have certain conditions, cutting meat can decrease your chances of clogged arteries, and eating burritos at a certain well-known fast food chain can increase your chances of spending the night on the toilet. I'm certainly not advocating that we all just say 'screw it' and start doing every unhealthy thing we've ever wanted to do as much as we want to do it, but I am saying that our choices aren't the only, or even necessarily the biggest, factor in our overall health. Yet, many people who are healthy act as if they have some secret that we don't.

There are people who've never once picked up a cigarette, but die of lung cancer. There are people who smoked every day up until their death, but never had a single health issue. Just because someone has never had a debilitating chronic illness, doesn't mean that they have the secret to healthy living or even that they will always be healthy. It's a fairytale that healthy people like to share to make them feel more secure and deserving of their healthiness, but it just isn't true.

Sometimes, people get sick through absolutely no fault of their own. Sometimes, we're handed a raw deal. Sometimes, you can make all the best choices and still end up sick. It's not our fault, and I've grown weary of healthy abled people who act like it is.

Bottom line...

We do not need someone with little to no understanding of our illnesses claiming that they know what will fix us. We do not need someone forcing us to justify our treatment plan. We do not need someone judging us for doing whatever is necessary for us to make it through the day. We do not need someone casting the blame of our illnesses on us. We do not need someone claiming that if we really wanted to be better, we would be, so we obviously are choosing to be sick.

What we do need is compassion, understanding, empathy, patience, and a willingness to learn more. My face lights up whenever a friend or family member tells me that they researched my illnesses to try to understand them better. Note: that feeling is immediately wiped away if they use a five-minute search to preach to me about what I should be doing. With all that we already have to deal with, toxic people with dangerous assumptions shouldn't be one of them.

IT'S OKAY NOT TO BE OKAY

"Mind over matter." "Just think positive thoughts." "Look on the bright side." These sayings are clichés for a reason. Positive thinking really can make a difference in how you feel and in your outlook on life. I am a big believer in the power of positivity, but....It's ok to not *always* feel positive.

Maybe this is already obvious to you and you're rolling your eyes while moving a finger flick towards the next essay in my book. But, maybe you're like me, where being positive has been drilled into you so much that you feel like a major failure when a bad day strikes that makes it difficult to see the silver lining.

Even as I write this piece, I feel like I'm somehow failing. I'm supposed to be happy and positive! I'm not supposed to share the secrets of my dark days. No one wants to hear about that crap, right?! But, that's exactly *why* we need to talk about it, because being sad doesn't mean you're failing. Because sadness is a normal human emotion and we're all allowed to feel it.

Sometimes a bad day will hit me out of nowhere. I'll go from feeling ok and even a little, dare I say, productive, to being in a full flare without the energy to lift my head. On those days, I have a hard time being optimistic. Why? The truth of the matter is, it freaking sucks. It just does. It sucks and it's not fair and it's not ok and I don't want to have to accept it. I want my old life back. Maybe I could've stayed all rainbows, sunshine, and lemonade had life actually given me lemons, but it didn't. It gave me incredibly painful, life altering illnesses and I don't really know how to make lemonade out of that.

I hate that I don't have a choice in this (other than my reaction, blah, blah, blah). I hate that I went from working full-time at a job I love, having great hobbies, actually seeing my friends, and feeling like a pretty good mom to suddenly having to redefine who I am in every single role I fill. I hate that a future that once seemed so tangible and clear has been ripped from me in a cruel and mystifying way. I hate that I have no idea what tomorrow will bring and that making plans often feels so pointless. I hate it all.

These aren't the days I typically blog about. On my worst days, I don't typically go running to Facebook to brag about how bad my attitude is or how long I sobbed into my pillow. I might fill Instagram with cynical comics on days like these, but I can't exactly post a picture of the weight that is bearing down on my soul. I have a feeling that this is pretty true of a lot of you reading this now. Sure, some people like to use social media as a therapist's couch, but a good majority of us try to stick to just the positive, happy highlights.

Now, I'm not suggesting that we all go the social-media-as-a-therapist's-couch route, but I am saying that an unrealistic picture is often painted, and we have to acknowledge that. Especially when it comes to people with chronic illnesses, be they physical or mental.

Every article or viral post about someone with an illness or a disability is talking about how strong they are because they choose to smile instead of cry. We're told that they refuse to let their illness get them down, and that this somehow makes them better than any other person with an illness. And yet, I guarantee you that even they have their "why me" days.

I believe that strength can be seen in many ways. There is strength in the woman who cries herself to sleep every night, but still finds something to smile about each morning. There is strength in a man who watches, with aching in his heart, countless others achieve the dream he can no longer reach but who also works to find another dream that is within his reach. There is strength in the child who spends all week angry at the universe for making him sick, but then still cheers on his former teammates as they play ball each weekend.

Being strong doesn't mean that you feel no pain. It doesn't mean that you never sob over the things you've lost, or long for the life you once had. Even the strongest of the strong have days where they can't stop crying or they want to give up.

Strength isn't the absence of dark days. Strength comes from getting back up, no matter how many times you break down. It comes from persevering even though you have no guarantee that things will get better. It comes from remembering that even your darkest of days don't define who you are and don't mean that you won't continue to fight. Feeling weak at different moments of your life doesn't make you a weak person.

When you live with chronic illness, you will grieve. You'll grieve for the life you dreamed of, the person you once were, the things you've had to give up. The world will try to tell you to tough it out, smile through it, look on the bright side, or be grateful that you don't have it worse…but they're wrong. It's great to be positive and grateful, and there's definitely a time and place for it, but you *have* to give yourself time to feel the hurt. Whenever we try to bottle up our emotions, they have a sneaky way of finding alternative ways to come out.

Grieving isn't a clean or linear process, especially with chronic illnesses. You may believe you've gotten through the worst of it, but then your favorite song comes on the radio and you can't sing along due to your illness and suddenly you're all the way back at Stage 1 of the grieving process. Or, you can be doing great and then a new symptom pops up that forces you to give up yet another thing you love and suddenly you're starting it all over again. There is no "getting over it." There's processing, acceptance, and moving forward, over and over again.

People believe that giving in to grief is a sign of weakness, but it truly takes great strength. Part of my treatment for PTSD (post-traumatic stress disorder) is to process the negative emotions attached to the trauma of my past, the emotions I've been trying to bury my entire life. That process has taught me just how much strength is required to truly feel the weight of that sorrow and to finally let it go.

Despite all the happy posts that flood social media, know that you aren't alone in your sadness. This grief comes with chronic illness. It's normal and natural, but because it's most often kept hidden, we feel completely alone in it. You're not. You're not alone. There are millions of us feeling these crushing and overwhelming feelings. Maybe it's time we start sharing them with each other, and walking this road together, so that the burden of it all can be a little lighter.

We are not failures because of our bad days. You are not a failure because of your bad days. Just try not to lose yourself in those bad days. Attempt to always fight your way back to the light, even if that means kicking, screaming, biting, and tearing your way back in. And, if you do feel lost in the darkness, talk to your doctor or other spoonies. Use every tool in your toolbox if you have to; you're much stronger than you know.

Love yourself, darkness and all.

SWEET CHILD OF MINE

Harper was barely 3-years-old when POTS came out of the woodwork and rendered me suddenly disabled. Most people struggle to remember things from before age six or seven. My earliest memories are from around five. That means that, barring some miracle cure for EDS and POTS, my daughter will really only remember me as her "sick" mommy.

She probably won't remember all the dance parties that she and I used to have, singing and spinning around the house. She won't remember the tickle fights or how I would lift her up to make her fly like an airplane. She won't remember how I used to drive her places while the two of us would sing at the top of our lungs. She won't remember all the meals I used to cook or all the times we would swing on the swings and slide down the slides. Instead, she'll remember me as the mommy who can't pick her up, who often has to sleep, who is always at the doctor, and who can't run and play with her anymore.

Her main memories of me will be of me and my illnesses. That's a heavy thought for me; however, that's because I still cling to the internalized belief that the old me was a better version of me. I mean, no doubt, being in less pain was certainly better, but I'm still a valuable human being. My value didn't decrease because I became disabled. Logically, I understand that and I preach it to all my fellow spoonies who struggle to see their own value.

Even so, I often beat myself up for the fact that I can't do all the things I used to be able to do with her, and that I can't teach her everything I'd hoped to teach her. However, that doesn't mean that I don't have valuable lessons that I can teach her. Reflecting on it, I think there are actually some pretty great lessons that she'll get to learn from me that are fairly unique to my struggles and disability:

Some people are disabled

Sure, that seems like a really obvious statement that no one should need a lesson on, and yet, our culture dismisses disabled people all the time. How many of the current shows on TV have disabled people in them? What about movies? How many shows or movies feature disabled people without a plot dedicated to them overcoming their disability?

Even when disabled characters do show up, they're usually poor representations of actual disabled people, as I've mentioned before. We're also only shown a very limited type of disability; most often, a paraplegic person in a wheelchair. We aren't shown various types of disabilities. Instead, we're shown that the person who uses the wheelchair in the store but then stands up in the parking lot is a faker and a con-man/con-woman. That's why citizens are proud to rush over to the girl, walking to her car in the disability parking spot, and scream in her face. They believe they are standing up for disabled people everywhere, because they don't understand that there are so many different types of disabilities.

My daughter will know. She'll know that disabilities come in all shapes and sizes. She'll know that, for some disabled people, they may have to use a rollator one day, walk on their own the next, and then end up in a wheelchair for a week. This is normal in her world. She won't be afraid or ashamed to look a person with a wheelchair in the eye when she's talking to them, unlike many able bodied adults. Harper will know how to treat us like the human beings we are, which is a lesson that a lot of people don't seem to have learned yet.

Compassion

Compassion is the ability to recognize that someone is suffering and having a desire to help relieve their suffering. It's a super important emotion that drives most charities and fundraisers. It swells in the heart of every passionate caretaker. It inspires people to take action against wrong doings and to march in the streets alongside marginalized groups, even if they themselves aren't marginalized.

The disability community needs people with compassion. We need doctors, nurses, hospital staff, social workers, lawyers, employers, friends, family, and even just random citizens, with compassion. We need people who will stand (or sit) with us as we fight for healthcare, accessibility, medical research, social security, and acceptance. We need people to love us and offer assistance without judgement when assistance is needed. This is, unfortunately, a very rare trait.

Through watching my struggle for healthcare, or experiencing difficulty getting into buildings that aren't up to ADA codes, or suffering from the cruel gaze of an unsympathetic stranger, I hope that Harper will develop such compassion. I hope that she will use that compassion to stand beside any group that is being marginalized and oppressed and help fight for their rights, because she has seen what it is like to be pushed aside and forgotten.

Empathy

Empathy is the ability to feel someone else's suffering. People often think that, to be truly empathetic, you have to have gone through the exact same situation. That's not true. It can be found by recognizing the emotion a person is feeling and remembering what that emotion feels like, even if the situation is different. It's seeing that someone is suffering and recognizing that you, too, have suffered.

You'll notice that the definition of empathy doesn't involve fixing problems in any way. Many of my problems can't be solved by anyone else, except maybe a doctor who stumbles upon a cure. For many people, it's a natural instinct to try to fix problems they see. But, no matter how good the intention, people telling me to try this supplement, or that doctor, or such and such diet, or whatever exercise…they aren't helping fix the problem. They are creating a whole new one.

While I know these suggestions come from a good place, they aren't what I need from people. I need people who will sit with me while I cry, who will agree with me when I say "this sucks" instead of telling me to "find the silver lining," who will stay beside me while I writhe in pain so that I don't have to be alone, who will laugh with me as we joke about ridiculous symptoms, and who'll listen to me when I just need to vent. I feel incredibly lucky to have people in my life who want to be able to fix my problems, but also recognize that they can't and will instead sit with me through the storm.

Harper's already begun to learn to do this. When I fainted in the kitchen one day, Harper came over to me and laid down next to me. We stayed there, talking together, until I was strong enough to stand up again. I see her ability to empathize grow more and more every day.

As much as I want to shield her from the darkest parts of my illnesses, I have a face that won't hide any of my emotions. And maybe that's a good thing. Maybe seeing the struggles as well as the good days will help her to become a more empathetic person. Maybe they will teach her how to sit with others as they ride out their own storms, because no one should feel like they are completely alone.

Sometimes you lose

A hard lesson to learn in life, one that no one really prepares you for: sometimes, even if you do everything right, you will still lose. We're taught that as long as you work really hard and stay the course, you'll eventually win. You may lose at first, but that's because you weren't working hard enough yet. It's all part of the great American "pull yourselves up by your bootstraps" dream that we've all heard over and over and over again.

Sometimes, no matter how hard we work for something or how much we want it, we won't get it. We will lose. Sometimes, no matter how well we take care of our bodies and how hard we try to stay healthy, we'll get sick and never get better.

It's scary to think about because it means we don't have control, but it's a reality. One of my favorite lines from *Jurassic Park* is when Laura Dern shouts out, "You never had control, that's the illusion!" Because, the truth is, a great majority of things in life *are* beyond our control.

Accepting that reality doesn't mean that we stop trying or stop working hard to achieve the things that we want, you definitely won't get what you want if you never try. It means that, if we do lose, we don't have to waste precious time and energy in feeling guilty for not being good enough. It also means that we stop assuming that people who aren't successful by our own standards are only that way due to lack of trying.

I want Harper to know that she should pursue her dreams with all she's got, but not waste time beating herself up if she doesn't get the life she thought she would have. She doesn't have to cling to a preconceived notion of success in order to be happy. If she loses, or gets sick, or meets any other hardships, that it's okay to let go of the old plan and start on something new. It's my hope for her that she will understand that sometimes bad things happen and there is no reason why. Sometimes the good guy loses, and that's okay. We keep trying anyway, we keep dreaming, but we don't waste time blaming ourselves.

To adapt, grow, and learn

Change is hard. Most of us struggle with accepting changes in our lives every now and then. Fear of change coupled with the idea that, if you keep at something, you'll eventually win, can sometimes be a very harmful combination. Determination in the face of adversity is great, unless you're running your head into a brick wall with the goal of breaking through.

When I first fell ill and became disabled, people kept telling me to stay strong and keep pushing through. I stubbornly held onto the idea that if I just worked hard enough, I'd eventually overcome all of my physical and mental limits to keep the life I had. Yet, if I had continued to push myself that way, I'm positive I would be in much worse health and I know that I wouldn't have had the strength or wherewithal to write this book.

This push to never change your focus, no matter what, comes from a survivor bias as well as a belief that we can't find happiness or purpose in multiple ways. The idea of each person only having one singular dream to chase is romantic, but extremely limiting. Sure, we've all heard stories of celebrities who lived in their cars or on the streets while pursuing their dream. We're told to worship that drive and mimic it in our own lives. What we don't see, is all the people who died waiting for something to happen that never did, who lived their life on hold while waiting for this elusive dream to come true.

Hard work, talent, determination…all of those are factors in success, but they aren't the only ones. I would hate to see Harper overlook options that could lead to a happy life simply because she believes that to change her mind is to give up. I don't want her to feel ashamed if one day, after years of chasing one dream, she decides that she doesn't want that dream anymore. I want her to know that happiness isn't a destination you reach once you've accomplished your goals, it's something you carry with you and bring into all that you do.

Not to judge the situations of others

Kinda along the lines of the "pull yourself up by your bootstraps," is the idea that anyone on any kind of government assistance shouldn't have anything of any kind of value. They shouldn't enjoy entertainment, take vacations, own technology, get new clothes, so on and so forth. It's like people expect those on assistance to live in cardboard boxes, use smoke signals for communication, dress in burlap sacks, wear shoes with holes in them, and walk everywhere they go. People of privilege have decided that people who require assistance are subhuman, because, after all, it is their fault that they are poor/unemployed/disabled/etc. since they obviously didn't work hard enough (see above).

The truth is, no one really knows what goes on in someone else's life unless they are living it. There are people who seem to foam at the mouth if they see a woman paying for her food with food stamps while she has an iPhone in her hand. Not only are they not considering that there are many reasons as to why the woman would have an iPhone and still need assistance, they are also not considering that it isn't actually any of their business. I've heard people declare, "If I have to pay for her food with my taxes then it's my business what she does with it." They seem to be under the impression that they are somehow owed proof of each persons' need. But that's not how taxes, communities, or life works. Just as they don't own a school because their taxes helped put it there, they don't own a person on assistance either.

My hope for Harper is that she'll know not to treat people like they're no longer people because they don't fit the picture society paints of what "poor," "disabled," or "in need" really looks like. I hope that she'll know that if she one day grows up to need government assistance, that she doesn't owe anyone an explanation and she isn't less of a human being because of it. Most importantly, I want her to know not to devalue *anyone's* existence just because she doesn't understand them.

What love looks like

We all know that movies and TV rarely get love and healthy relationships right. But, until I fell in love with Matt, I didn't realize which parts were wrong. My first marriage often resembled these fictional relationships, because it was full of big dramatic fights and lots of drama. Everyone was always preaching about how hard relationships are, so I assumed it was all normal. What I assumed was made up was how two people could be lovers, partners, and best friends. I was sure that the respect, care, desire, and excitement fictional couples felt was all exaggerated. The real thing, in my experience, was much more lackluster.

Then came Matt.

Our relationship isn't the stuff they'd write movies or books about, but that's not because of a lack of love. It's because conflict is what sells a story, and we've had little of that when it comes to the two of us. There are no big messy break-up scenes that are followed by chases through the airport and public declarations of love. We don't get into weekly spats over absurd things that often involve lying, vengeance, and studio audience laughter. Our story would certainly seem boring to most, but the love felt is deeper than I ever thought possible.

That's not to say we have an easy life or that we never argue. On the contrary, our life has been very messy and difficult, thanks to my new chronic illnesses. Chaos, drama, and tragedies have swirled around us over the years, but we've faced each and every one of them together. We were put to the "in sickness and in health" test fairly early on in our relationship, and so far it's only brought us closer.

Now, our relationship is still relatively young. We have a whole lot more growing to do and mountains to face, but I've never been in a relationship where I felt even a fraction of the love and security we have now. I just never knew it was possible. But Harper will. She'll grow up knowing that sometimes, when in the midst of the darkness, love can be your greatest ally.

Alright, alright, I know it sounds like I'm bragging, or that we're in some unrealistic love bubble that'll soon pop. It's hard for me to explain how amazed I am by the beautiful healthy ordinariness of it all. There are no big fancy gifts, surprise cross country trips, or any grand gestures like that. It's the homemade presents, prescriptions that are picked up, knowing how I take my coffee, and all the laughter. That's our love. Thousands of little things that go undetected by onlookers, but mean the world to us. And that's the kind of love I hope Harper will find for herself one day.

To be a warrior

Earlier, I detailed some of the different ways that I fight daily. I fight for what I need. I fight for what I want. I fight for what I have. I fight for all that I've lost. Every day is a battle of some kind; there isn't a single day where I don't have to be a warrior in order to keep living life.

Facing daily battles requires great strength and resilience. I've been knocked down more times than I can count, and yet I keep getting back up. I've had to start over, change plans, and let go of things I fought to have. It's devastating to put your heart, blood, and soul into something only to see it slip through your fingers, but I've done it more than once. Through all of this, I've learned that there is no one way to be strong, or brave, or tough. There's no one way to keep fighting. What matters most, and is perhaps the biggest struggle of them all, is staying true to myself no matter how the battle rages on.

I don't know what the future holds for my daughter. I don't know if she'll have an easy life, where things just seem to fall into place for her, or if she'll have mountains to move. EDS is genetic, so she has a 50% chance of having it. Even if she does have it, we have no way of knowing if it will affect her the way I'm affected. It could be better, it could be worse. Whether she breezes through life or faces daily struggles, I hope that she'll take strength with her in whatever she does. I hope that, no matter the obstacles in her path, she not only fights for herself, but for others as well.

Lastly, I want for her to remember what all the fighting is for, because it's really easy to forget when you're stuck in the thick of it. Despite all the ugliness of the world, there's a lot of beauty as well. There's goodness, laughter, love, kindness, generosity, connections, adventures, wonder, and magic all around. Finding these things within all the chaos, hatred, and oppression is a war all of its own, but it's one that I hope to never stop fighting. Because, to me, those are the things that make it all worth it. Yes, I'm a whimsical, romantic, bleeding heart, softy…and I fight hard to stay that way. I hope Harper will, too.

THE HIGH COST OF SPOONIE LIVING

My husband and I just finished our monthly discussion of our household finances. Well, it's really more of a ritual discussion of our lack of funds and a run-down of different possibilities to prepare for, including, but not limited to: praying to the gods of money, planting some pennies to see if they grow money trees, or running into the social security office shouting, "will somebody please approve my disability case!" I'll keep you posted on how those ideas turn out.

As I just bragged about in the previous essay, Matt truly is my partner in life. Since POTS hit, he has taken on extra duties in our life, such as: preparing all the meals, doing almost all shopping, driving everyone where they need to go, playing with our daughter while I rest, packing her lunches, getting school supplies, taking her shopping for clothes, picking up my prescriptions, and many other things I'm forgetting that he'll remind me of later. I think of myself as incredibly lucky to have him, not because I'm a burden or less deserving of a good partner, but because he truly makes my life better in every way.

As you can see, taking care of both Harper and I is practically a full-time job in itself. On top of that, Matt works absurd hours at an entry level position, paying his dues to get better positions, as well as part-time online work that he's able to do from home. I'm not sharing this so you regard him as a saint, or take pity on us, but, rather, to help paint a picture of the cost of life with chronic illnesses.

When Matt and I first moved in together, he had just finished school and was starting on his new career. I was finishing my Master's degree while also beginning my career as a full-time lead teacher. We didn't make much, but we managed, and were even able to tuck funds away into savings in the hopes of one day being able to put it towards a down payment on a house. It seemed that we were on a clear path upward.

Then came POTS.

Obviously, our family budget changed once I had to step down from my job, but even before I had to leave, we were suddenly facing a new expense none of us could have predicted. Just in the first few months of my diagnosis, I had paid over $4,000 in medical expenses on top of my insurance premium. Thank God for the ACA's yearly out of pocket limits, because I have met mine by March of the past few years.

Once my salary dropped exponentially, I discovered that I no longer qualified for subsidies since I fell into the needs-Medicaid-but-only-if-your-state-expanded category. My state is not an expansion state, which means they sent me a lovely letter explaining how I didn't make enough for subsidies, but I don't really deserve Medicaid, so instead they'll just wave the fee for not being insured. That's not very helpful when you *have* to have insurance for you multiple chronic illnesses.

That first year of zero subsidy insurance, I'd accrued a whopping $8,000 in medical bills (minus the premium I paid out of savings and couldn't afford) by March. You may be asking, "How does someone accrue $8,000 in medical expenses within a few months without a major surgery or cancer?" Well, actually, you may not be asking that question if you are a US citizen, because most of us recognize how expensive even routine medical care is. My medications alone (all of which are required for me to be even somewhat functional) total well over $1,000 a month. Newer medications, fresh on the market, are the worst for the lining of your wallets. One such medicine, which has helped keep my flares from being as severe and lasting as long, is $500 a month with no generic options.

There were medicines I needed but had to stop taking until I met my out-of-pocket limit just because I couldn't afford to pay for them. Add to that $200 for each specialist visit (at least two a month), $500 for a bag of IV fluids at an urgent care center, two months of physical therapy, and three ER visits due to crashing vitals, and it's pretty easy to see how quickly it all adds up.

This is where I'd like to point out, for anyone thinking "well, duh, that's traditional medicine for you," that going the nontraditional route is anything but affordable. We've had to get creative with meal planning due to my various dietary restrictions, as healthier foods tend to be more expensive. We try to eat whole foods whenever possible, but there's also the disappointing feeling when your fresh fruits and veggies go bad because you were too nauseous to eat anything but saltines for half the week. I had a blood panel done to see what vitamins and nutrients my body needed help supplementing. In return I got a list of at least $500 worth of monthly supplements, none of which would actually replace my medicines. Even just a visit with a holistic specialist is expensive, but doesn't have the added bonus of at least going towards the deductible.

Another little known fact is that many "alternative" healthcare providers won't take on patients with severe chronic illnesses, or will only take you on in addition to you still seeing a regular healthcare provider. I have had multiple alternative care professionals express that they either could not take me on, or wouldn't be comfortable working with me without a relationship with my specialists, just because of the nature and scope of my illnesses. A chiropractor, acupuncturist, personal trainer, nutritionist, massage therapist...all of those may be able to help some with my symptoms, but they can't cure me. So, they become additional costs to my already too expensive healthcare.

It should not be taken for granted that alternative healthcare is not a viable option for many chronically ill people. Please stop shaming people for using every tool available to them to fight their illnesses, rather than just the ones you think they should use. I cannot say this enough, unless you are a doctor who is intimately familiar with our medical history, do not tell us how we can "cure" incurable illnesses or that the only reason we're still sick is because we aren't trying hard enough to be well. I cannot over emphasize how incredibly harmful that attitude is. It absolutely does not help anyone to get better.

Within 20 months of being diagnosed, our income has been reduced by at least half, and we have taken on the financial equivalent of adding a second child to our home. We have watched our savings go from a healthy promise, to a teasing wink. I have been incredibly fortunate to find another part time job working from home, and Matt is on track for a promotion at his job. We're also still waiting to get a hearing for disability benefits. We remain hopeful for better days to come, and we cover each other in love and kindness every single day. But, we still walk around with the weight of knowing that at any given moment I could end up needing expensive surgeries, or hospital stays, or more diagnostic tests, or any myriad of possibilities. We have seen how quickly everything can change, for better or worse.

The cruel irony is that, regardless of how much we planned for the future or how much effort we put into bettering our lives, now that I'm disabled, there are people who treat us like we're lazy and just looking for handouts. It's as if some people come with an empathy expiration date. They felt badly when they saw our circumstances changing, but now think that it's obviously our fault that things haven't gotten better. It's back to that whole "if you tried harder" mentality I've ranted about before.

Now, everything we do is held up under a magnifying glass, as certain people search for ways to blame us for our own situation. If we just worked harder, if I just wanted to feel better, if we just got better jobs, if we just stopped spending money (who needs electricity?), or if we had just planned better, then apparently we wouldn't be in the situation we are now. People will jump through hoops just to find a way to point the finger at someone else and absolve themselves of any social responsibility.

I think it's hard for some healthy people to understand the toll that chronic illness takes on a person's bank account. Many people boil it down to the cost of insurance, which is in itself out of reach for so many people, but they don't realize how quickly the copays, prescriptions, tests, medical devices, and supplemental items add up and steal any glimmer of financial security a person may have felt. They don't realize how hard it is to try and dig yourself out of a pit of debt when that pit is growing larger and larger by the minute.

We're lucky. I know that sounds odd considering all that I've written above, but truly we're lucky. We have a savings to drain and family members who're willing to help us out. We started off fairly stable, not well-off by any stretch, but able to pay all our bills with a little left over to spare. We had created a cushion, one that is barely a sliver of fabric now, but it still has helped keep us from crashing. Not everyone is so lucky.

People die every day waiting to receive disability benefits. People die because they can't afford lifesaving medical treatment. I, myself, have turned down an ambulance even when I was in dire need because I couldn't afford the cost. I've had to decide whether I should get my medicines for the month or be able to pay a bill on time. And then, we are blamed for our struggles and told that we don't deserve healthcare/medications/water/whatever because we just aren't trying hard enough.

I've been in some ugly debates about government assistance and healthcare. I've had people straight up tell me that if I was too sick to work then it was nature's way of saying I'm not supposed to live. I've been told that I'm a burden and that it should be up to each individual citizen to decide if they want to help others out or not, that it shouldn't be mandatory through taxes. Honestly, I just don't understand the argument.

I don't understand how some lives are decided to be more valuable than others based on a person's financial status. I can't wrap my head around the idea that it's ok for people to die because they can't afford the medical bill. And I really don't get why some people think that it's acceptable to charge sick people more money for the same product, like insurance, meaning that only the wealthy can get adequate care.

Chronic illnesses are far more expensive than people realize. My illnesses cost me my job, my savings, my social life, my independence, and my dreams. In the eyes of many people, it also cost me my core value as a human being. It cost me my right to healthcare and other basic necessities. It cost me my right to live.

If you can't work, you are still valuable. If you have chronic illness or illnesses, you are still valuable. If you have disabilities, you are still valuable. If you are gay/straight/bi/trans/black/white/world citizen/any other qualifier you can think of...You. Are. Valuable. And you are deserving of all the fundamental rights afforded to every other human being.

Chronic illnesses cost us a lot of things, but that shouldn't be one of them.

JUST SAY 'NO' TO INSPIRATION PORN

There's a strange phenomenon on the internet that we, in the disability community, refer to as "inspiration porn." The general idea of this is where abled people use pictures of disabled people to exclaim how inspirational they are simply for existing, or using it to guilt abled people into trying harder because if a *disabled* person can brush their teeth, then surely *you* can do anything.

In the interest of full disclosure, before I became disabled, I didn't realize how harmful this was. I fully admit that I participated in perpetuating this. I'm positive I shared a viral inspiration porn post at some point in time, and used it to inspire me to push harder. So, understand that this post isn't to vilify people for taking part in inspiration porn but, rather, to show people how harmful it actually is so that you can learn to do better. In other words, don't get pissed off at me for calling it out if this is something you do. Take a deep breath, and take on a new perspective.

Why is inspiration porn harmful? Well, for one, having a disability or chronic illness does not automatically make you a morally righteous person. For instance, Oscar Pistorious, known as the 'Blade Runner,' is a disabled man who was convicted of murdering his girlfriend.

Evil comes in all shapes, sizes, colors, and abilities. Disability doesn't equal morality.

Continuing on, inspiration porn objectifies disabled people. It's absolutely wonderful to celebrate the accomplishments of disabled people, just as it is to celebrate the accomplishments of abled people. However, when images of disabled people are accompanied by slogans such as, "what's your excuse?" or "your excuse is invalid" disabled people aren't being lifted up or celebrated. We're being used as a tool to guilt abled people into trying harder.

Images like that ignore the fact that there are many different types of disabilities and perpetuate the assumption that disabled people shouldn't be able to do anything. This just is not true. Take the all-too popular pictures of people running with prosthetic limbs saying something like "never give up" or "you can do it." The disabilities of the people in those pictures happen to allow them to run with the help of aids. I don't need prosthetic limbs, but my disability keeps me from running due to wild heart rate fluctuations and dizziness. If my mind didn't give up on running, my body certainly would.

Yet, the effect of these images leads people to say things such as, "well, did you see that picture of the little boy with no legs who competed on a track team? He's disabled and can still do stuff like that, so why can't you?" Well, Brenda, because we have different kinds of disabilities which allows us to do different types of activities, so stop telling me that I can climb the stairs if I just 'believe' and let me use the damn elevator!

Inspiration porn puts pressure on disabled people to think that they have to be an "inspiration" to matter. It's not enough to live our lives and learn how to work with our disabilities, we also have to inspire millions of abled people to recognize how "lucky" they are to be abled. It sends the message that if a disabled person is capable of completing simple tasks, then abled people should be able to do 1000 times better. It's like saying, "hey, watch out abled peeps, disabled people are accomplishing things which makes them look equal to us, so we need to work harder because we're obviously better and more capable than they are at everything." Yes, *everything*. I have seen images of a disabled person getting dressed accompanied with the message of "what's your excuse," because, apparently, abled people are also supposed to be better at getting dressed than disabled people.

Telling me that I'm an inspiration because I brushed my teeth isn't encouraging. It's infantilizing and demeaning. I want to inspire people with my words or my determination in fighting for the rights of all people, not by the fact that I managed a grin on a tough day. If we're told we're inspiring for every small insignificant thing, then it's like we're being told that there are no greater expectations of us, as if no disabled person has ever changed the world. Be inspired by the fact that I wrote a book, because that's damn inspiring if I say so myself, not by the fact that I manage to wake up every morning. Don't set my bar so low.

Another popular trope for inspiration porn is that abled people are heroes simply for treating disabled people like human beings. Disabled people date. We have sex. We fall in love. We get married. We have kids. These things aren't happening in spite of our conditions, our conditions are part of us. Had Matt slipped, "I take you to be my wife, even though you're disabled" into his vows, I probably would've rolled my disabled ass right back down that aisle. No one gets brownie points for being friends or lovers with disabled people. And if they are only hanging out with disabled people to get said brownie points, then they aren't actually good people.

Being disabled doesn't make someone unworthy of love. When people share images of a kid all dressed up in a wheelchair standing next to an abled person with the line "even though she has a disability, he still took her to prom" all it does is tell disabled people that we aren't worthy of basic human decency. It tells us that our disabilities are seen as inherently bad and undesirable. It tells us that our disabilities are things that someone has to look past in order to love us.

That's a really crappy message to send out.

My disability is part of me. It's part of who I am. I can't shed it or put it aside, not even for a moment. It's not something shameful or embarrassing that someone has to look past. Most importantly, it doesn't make me any less human or deserving of kindness. This belief is one of the many reasons why disabled people are far more likely to be in abusive relationships. When the world is constantly telling you that you're lucky if someone even smiles at you, then you start to believe you have to take what you can get, no matter how awful it might be.

And, finally, perhaps the most harmful of all the effects of inspiration porn, is the notion that our lives aren't worth living. When someone tells a disabled person "you are so inspiring, I don't know how you do it, I couldn't live like that," they are telling us that they see our life as miserable and unworthy. They are telling us that they can't believe we haven't killed ourselves because they couldn't imagine ever living the way we live. People constantly telling you that they think your life is horrible starts to get under your skin. And it can start to make you question whether or not they're right.

Wading through a sea of messages telling me that my life is unworthy doesn't make me feel strong or brave for living it, it makes me feel like my life isn't valued by the message sender. Believe me, I hate being sick. I hate having constant pain. I hate having to face new limitations that get in the way of what I used to be able to do. But, I absolutely believe my life is worth living. I am fortunate enough to have an amazing life partner and feisty daughter. I have an awesome support group of friends, both online and face-to-face. I have things that I'm passionate about and I'm finding ways to continue to do them, in one way or another. And I love who I am as a person, and that includes my disability.

I firmly believe that everyone has the potential to be inspiring. Throughout history, there have been many great inspirers who helped bring about great change. There are also those who inspire others on a smaller scale: teachers who inspire students to learn, coaches who inspire their players to pick themselves up after a loss, activists who inspire others to take up the cause…Yet, not all teachers, coaches, or activists are inspirational. If they were, then there wouldn't be anything special about the ones who truly incite change, either in the world or in someone's heart.

My hope has always been to inspire people. But, if I'm told that I'm inspiring simply for being alive, then it makes it feel like all my hard work has been for nothing. And when abled people use me as some kind of reminder to be grateful or as some litmus test for what an abled person should be able to do, it hurts me. It tells me that neither my life nor my skills are valued.

I think most people mean well when they share these things, which is why I think calling it out is so important. We need to challenge each other to be better, to *do* better. Disabled people all over are being hurt in very real ways because of this trend, so it really has to stop. There are plenty of things to be inspired by out in the real world, my disability doesn't need to be one of them.

TRIGGERED

Every year, for Independence Day in the good ole US of A, neighborhoods across the country have fireworks, big ones, going off all night for at least three days before the 4th and at least three days after. In the past few years, I've started to see signs making their way around social media. Signs that read "A veteran lives here, please be respectful with your fireworks." I've seen people share these images with pride and remind everyone how important it is to think of combat veterans during this time.

These signs are typically placed in front of the houses of veterans with Post Traumatic Stress Disorder (PTSD) and they are essentially reverse trigger warnings. Now, I love seeing people share this image and remind others to be mindful of the mental health of those around them, but I also find it interesting that many of the people sharing images like this one are the same people who make fun of trigger warnings used in articles, posts, images, etc.

Perhaps interesting isn't the right word there...frustrating, that seems more accurate. I've seen many people rant about how sensitive everyone is nowadays that there are trigger warnings on everything. People who need or use trigger warnings are called "snowflakes" and told that we're basically just a bunch of big babies. The term "triggered" is flung around as an insult and used to describe anyone with any kind of emotional reaction. Honestly, I don't know where all the animosity comes from, but I'm gonna give people the benefit of the doubt and assume that maybe it comes from a misunderstanding of what trigger warnings really are and what purpose they serve.

I have PTSD. No, I've never served in the military or seen a day of combat. Unlike the general accepted belief, not everyone with PTSD has done those things. I have a specific type of PTSD called C-PTSD, or Complex PTSD. For me, it comes from prolonged childhood trauma as well assault. Thanks to EDS and POTS, I also have an over-reactive sympathetic nervous system which can cause adrenaline surges from even the smallest amounts of stimulation. I am a person who needs trigger warnings.

Trigger warnings are like yield signs for people with PTSD. They tell me, "Hey, this could potentially trigger your past trauma and cause you to spiral into the depths of anxiety and depression." It gives me the option to weigh the risks and benefits of a TV show, movie, activity, book, article, social media post, etc. I need trigger warnings if a video is going to be really loud, bright, or include jump scares, because those will set off my sympathetic nervous system. If I accidently stumble upon a post describing sexual assault, abuse, or death in great detail, it will trigger my PTSD. Trigger warnings help me feel more secure and in control. Without them, the world, especially the internet, becomes a much scarier place.

Some of the misunderstandings about trigger warnings might stem from people not understanding what it actually means to be triggered. I've seen it used to mean offended, angry, sad, shocked, unhappy, or any slightly negative emotion. Perhaps there are some people who use trigger warnings in that way, but that is not their intention.

Being triggered means that something has aggravated my PTSD which leaves me with feeling as if the trauma is happening all over again right then and there. Just like how loud fireworks can trigger a flashback to combat for a veteran, it can trigger a flashback of abuse for me. I don't literally see it happening or lose track of where I am, but my mind goes back to it. It's not me being overly dramatic, it's my brain chemistry.

My mind and body remember what the original trauma felt like and reacts as if it's happening all over again. I can be sitting comfortably at home and all of a sudden I'll feel as if I'm in imminent danger. My heartrate will shoot right up and I end up nauseated, dizzy, lightheaded, scared, and terribly sad. It can take hours, days, or even weeks to recover from one triggering episode. When all of that happens because I accidentally stumbled upon a video with triggering content, it can be infuriating.

This isn't something that I have any power over. I don't get to choose what is triggering to me and what isn't. I can't just turn it off and decide that it's no longer upsetting. As a survivor of assault, when a man who bragged openly about sexual assault was elected president, I immediately was thrown back into all those feelings attached to my own assault. It hit me out of nowhere. I felt as though I had just been punched in the gut. I couldn't stop crying and felt unsafe everywhere I went. As I was grappling with all of these feelings, I was also trying to understand where it came from and why it happened. While I was unhappy with the latest presidential election results, I didn't expect that it would trigger my PTSD.

I'm sure some of you are rolling your eyes right about now, and no you can't have your money back that you spent on this book. I'm simply trying to illustrate how sometimes the things that trigger us are just as much of a surprise to us as it is to other people. I'm not suggesting that there should be a giant trigger warning placed before all election results, nor am I saying that I was triggered merely because my candidate lost. What I'm trying to do is to show how being triggered isn't something we choose to do. In fact, the whole reason I want trigger warnings is so I can avoid that feeling whenever possible.

PTSD doesn't care about logic and it doesn't care about intentions. Someone telling me, "I didn't mean it like that, you just need to get over it," doesn't stop my mind from reliving the trauma. Someone saying, "But it's not really happening again, you're safe, so why does it bother you," will also have zero effect on my PTSD. I have many methods to try to cope with an attack, including grounding myself, but I can't logic my way out of them. It's an odd and incredibly exasperating feeling to know that logically there is no reason for you to be upset, but your brain just won't listen.

Here's the thing I think a lot of people are failing to realize: You don't have to understand why something is triggering to me for it to be triggering. Just as able bodied people tend to demand for disabled people to prove their disability, those without mental illness often demand explanations for our reactions. Only when they are reactions that they can understand will they then decide that our reactions are valid. But, my PTSD doesn't care if you understand it or not, it exists all the same.

Many people who scoff at trigger warnings don't hesitate to jump all over someone who says that they've been triggered. They'll feverishly type out comments like "you're an idiot if that bothers you," or "well, I would be triggered by the opposite thing," or "you need to lighten up." I can't really stress enough how unhelpful these comments are and how they, again, won't change the fact that I've been triggered.

I've also found that some people get really offended at being told that something they've posted could be triggering and might need a trigger warning. They'll stomp and shout about First Amendment rights and how I'm trying to eliminate freedom of speech. I'm not saying that people should be dragged out of their homes and tossed into prison cells for putting up a triggering post. I'm asking for a little understanding and consideration.

So, yes, trigger warnings matter. They matter to my mental health and well-being. No, the world will never be trigger proof and it's not anyone's job to bubble wrap all the mental sharp edges that may be out there. However, if doing something as simple as adding a warning to a possibly triggering post could help make someone's life easier, why wouldn't someone want to do it? Accessibility is rarely as easy as adding a couple words to the opening of a post, so why is there so much pushback? It's not about differing opinions or free speech, it's about respect for other people. It's about taking one small step towards making the world a better place. So, let's do it.

MY BODY AND ME

I have struggled with body image my entire life. Unfortunately, in our society, that is not an uncommon statement. In fact, we tend to find it unusual when someone says, "I love my body, I always have." However, my body image issues went beyond the socially acceptable stereotype of the woman who perpetually wants to lose 15 lbs.

I didn't just have poor body image, I had body loathing. I spent the better part of my life feeling like I was a hideous monster that no one could possibly ever love. I remember standing in the kitchen at age twelve grabbing, pinching, and tugging on the unacceptable parts of my body, wishing that I could hack them off with a kitchen knife. Maybe then I'd be worthy of love.

In my teens, this negative image of myself was reinforced by those around me, which only made my self-loathing seem more appropriate. Everyone fawns over the slender beautiful girl who says she's hideous, but when a chubby awkward girl says it, there's usually a painful silence followed by: "have you tried dieting," "at least you have a pretty face," or "you're pretty, just in a weird way." Self-hatred is expected if you don't fit into the societal image of an acceptable body.

Nowadays, body image is a popular topic. We, as a society, talk about fat shaming and unrealistic body expectations. While some progress has been made, we've still got a long way to go. I've seen people defending body shaming because "being overweight is unhealthy and we shouldn't let people think that it's ok." Yes, it's true that being overweight can cause a lot of health problems. But, sometimes health problems are what cause someone to be overweight. Sometimes, a person can be overweight, yet still be in great health. Sometimes, a person can be thin and have health problems. Basically, a person's body type isn't always indicative of their health.

Even if weight was an automatic indicator of health, that doesn't make body shaming okay. What so many people are failing to see is that body positivity isn't about embracing unhealthy habits. It's about not hating yourself because of the girth of your waist. It's about knowing that there is so much more to you than your pant size. And, it's about understanding that your value as a human being does not stem from the numbers on a scale.

Body positivity also goes beyond weight. Magazines, movies, TV, and other forms of media all promote a very narrow definition of beautiful. More often than not, the desirable person is white, thin, and able bodied. There usually are very few scars, tattoos, piercings, or prosthetics. Anyone who doesn't fit into that mold is either airbrushed into conformity or left out altogether. These narrow standards make it difficult for anyone to love their body when they don't fit in. That's what body positivity is working against. It's telling people that no matter what you look like, you should still love yourself.

I've told myself these things at least a thousand times. I've given myself countless pep talks. I truly, in my heart, believe all of it. It's my eyes that need to catch up. And now that I have chronic illnesses, where it feels like my body is actively fighting against me every single day, I'm finding it even harder to love myself, cellulite and all.

Here's where I need to make a confession. It's something I thought about writing a million different posts for, but I never found the courage to put it down on paper until now. Maybe knowing that it will live within the pages of my very own book is what has pushed me to open up. Or, maybe it's the fact that there is no comment section at the bottom of this page, so I don't have to worry about it immediately being tossed in my face.

On top of all of my conditions, I also struggle with a chronic mental affliction: an eating disorder. It's something that never leaves me, no matter how hard I try to shut it out. I haven't "acted out" in my eating disorder in a very long time, but that doesn't mean I'm cured. It still whispers in my ear about how I'm not good enough and undeserving of love. It taps me on the shoulder to tell me how revolting I am as I stand in front of the mirror. And it shouts at me that I'm a failure whenever I struggle to button my pants.

Most people have misconceptions about eating disorders. It's not as simple as crash dieting, and doesn't go away when you reach a certain weight. In fact, when I finally found my way to the road to recovery, I was under a healthy weight for my body and yet, I still saw myself as some creature of the deep. The truth is that eating disorders are addictions and they aren't really about the weight. They are about what you attach to the weight. For me, it was love.

I believed that if I looked a certain way, all of my problems would be solved. If I was a certain size, then people who had hurt me would finally love and accept me. I would no longer feel like an outcast. I would no longer feel all alone. And yet, no matter how much my appearance changed, this magic feeling of happiness and satisfaction never came, which only made me dive deeper into my disorder.

Recovery from an eating disorder is anything but easy. It's a battle I fight daily, along with all the other wars waging on inside my body. But, I have come a very long way. Or, I had, until my chronic illnesses hit.

Before proceeding, let me first tell you about the one really amazing year where I actually loved my body and all that it could do:

It started when I left my ex-husband and the marriage that seemed to be devouring me little by little until I couldn't recognize the person in the mirror anymore. I had spent the year leading up to our separation trying to find myself again, or for the first time, I suppose. I wanted to figure out where the real me had been hidden away and if she still had any life in her. That journey continued on after I left. I felt like a prisoner finally being released from their cage: free and seeing the world all over again with brand new eyes.

I began an intense yoga regimen. I did yoga as much as I could wherever I could. I wasn't doing it with the goal of changing my appearance. Rather, I was doing it because it felt good. I felt centered and grounded all at once. I ate as clean as possible. I meditated daily. And, because of all of that, I suddenly felt at one with my body. My dualistic view of "me" vs "my body" melted away and gently fused together. I was my body and it was me. We were no longer enemies working against each other.

I had never in my life felt so free and connected. Strength radiated from my pores. I didn't care about clothing size, weight, or how I looked. I felt comfortable in my own skin, a feeling I was in no way used to or prepared for. While I now know that I still had undiagnosed Ehlers-Danlos syndrome, the exercises helped tamp down the symptoms. I had fewer injuries, less joint pain, and slept deeper than ever before. I felt like an entirely different person.

But, then, as you know, POTS hit and rendered me disabled. I could no longer do yoga because the positional changes caused me to pass out. I tried doing simple floor exercises but my heart rate would shoot up dangerously high with the smallest amount of activity. My energy stores were limited anyway and I chose to use what energy I had on my job and family rather than using it all up for yoga. I tried various other exercises with similar results, but nothing helped. Every time I would get into an exercise routine and start building my strength again, a new symptom or injury would emerge, knocking me back down again.

My body had betrayed me, or that's how it felt. I had spent a year treating it like a temple and now it had given out on me. It was no longer part of me but, rather, an enemy trying to steal away every ounce of who I was.

In the time since my diagnosis, the numbers on the scale have increased. I've watched my lean muscles turn soft and begin to sag. I have a closet full of clothes I can no longer wear and a stack of expensive compression leggings that went from difficult to impossible to put on. I am once again struggling with body image and the fear that, as everything else I've known has been slipping away, my own body is slipping away from me as well.

How am I supposed to love a body that seems intent on destroying me? How can I take care of a body that keeps beating me down?

Perhaps the answer lies in how I view my illnesses as well as my body. I tend to think of my illnesses as belonging to my body. They are part of my genetic make-up, after all. But, what if I thought about my illnesses as something separate from my body? As invaders who forced their way in and now are refusing to leave? Maybe, instead of my body and I being enemies, we're allies, fighting the damage of the intruders together.

Or, maybe I need to stop thinking about my body or my illnesses as being evil. If I can truly accept my illnesses for what they are, accept my limitations, and accept my needs, then it won't feel as though my body is constantly under attack. It's when I think of all the things I 'should' be doing that I become the most frustrated with myself. I think that maybe it's time for me to let go of the 'shoulds' and focus on the 'cans.'

I refuse to continue to hate my body. It feels like living in an inescapable prison, with no option of parole. I hope to get to where I can exercise regularly again, and I'd love to see my lean muscles come back, but I know that I can't depend on those things for loving my body. I have to stop hating it now. I have to, or it's going to tear me apart.

My body may be soft, but that doesn't mean I'm not strong.

ACCESSIBILITY NOW

In 1990, the Americans with Disabilities Act (ADA) was passed into law. It is a piece of civil rights legislation that makes it illegal to discriminate against anyone with a disability in all aspects of public life: meaning jobs, health care, schools, transportation, and any public or private facility that is open to the general public. Disabled Americans fought hard for this bill, many being arrested and brutalized in hopes of its passing. One of the hallmarks of this bill was accessibility. Any public building without wheelchair access is automatically discriminatory against disabled people, as it isn't open for disabled people to get to.

Before I became disabled, I assumed that the ADA fixed all accessibility issues. Since becoming disabled, I've learned just how wrong I was. I also never realized that there were people who are against the ADA. I learned about it as the House and Senate were voting on a bill that would weaken the ADA. I couldn't imagine anyone thinking that accessibility was a bad thing, but lo and behold, I quickly found myself in multiple debates with people telling me that businesses shouldn't have to cater to my needs.

An argument that those against the ADA use is that

it's an expensive burden on small businesses. I was told that it's unreasonable to ask small businesses to pay to be accessible to everyone. I was told that the government shouldn't have a say in how a business conducts itself, and that profits should drive a company to be accessible or not. Essentially, the ADA was positioned as being oppressive to small business owners rather than a protection of the civil rights of disabled people.

This debate points to a much larger issue. It shows how acceptable ableism still is, the belief that disabled people are burdens, and a grave misunderstanding as to what accessibility really is and why it matters.

First, let's talk about life before the ADA. The world was largely inaccessible, which left many disabled people living in group homes under subpar care, simply because it was their only option. Investigations into such homes revealed them to be abusive and neglectful, but disabled people didn't have access to public buildings, school, or work, which left them without any alternatives.

Not only did the ADA make it so workplaces can't discriminate based on ability for hiring, but now the buildings had to be accessible as well. This is better in theory than in practice, as many places refuse to become fully accessible. I mean, it's pretty easy to say, "We don't discriminate in our hiring process" while simultaneously being inaccessible to disabled people, showing how actions truly do speak louder than words. When it comes to disabilities, discrimination is seen not only in prejudiced behavior, but also in denial of access.

Second, let's talk about life with the ADA. It absolutely is a whole lot better than life before the ADA, that's for sure, but there are still many obstacles (literal and figurative) that disabled people face daily. The world around us is still largely inaccessible. Unfortunately, it's not really a problem most people notice until they have to. Yet, when you're disabled, it's impossible to ignore.

For instance, the ADA states that all places need to be accessible to enter. Many places have accessible entrances, or alternative entrances, for this very purpose. However, once you're inside they aren't really accessible at all. Often, it's hard to move around in your wheelchair or with your mobility device, or there will be steps that lead to different parts of the inside of the building. I went to a restaurant one time where there was a ramp to get in, but the bathrooms were down a large flight of stairs. I had to have someone walk up and down the stairs with me, to help support me, so that I wouldn't pass out along the way. It would have been near impossible if I was on my own. It absolutely is impossible for many other disabled people.

Since becoming disabled, I have discovered what a nightmare accessibility truly is even with the ADA. I have encountered ramps too steep to push myself up, and almost too steep for Matt to push me . I've seen ramps that inexplicably lead to a step. There are ramps that are ridiculously far from the front entrance, not a huge problem if I'm being pushed in my wheelchair, but almost impossible if I'm trying to push myself or am using my rollator.

One frustrating case was when we went to a park, which cost us $45 per person to enter, which claimed to have disability accessibility. Once inside the park, we discovered that the accessible part of the park was one small path that went from the entrance to a scenic view in the back. That's it. None of the attractions or exhibits were actually accessible, yet we were charged full price for the ticket. Honestly, I'm still peeved about it. Fellow disabled people, beware of Lookout Mountain Park in Chattanooga, Tennessee. Their accessibility is a joke.

Annoyance quickly turned to downright dangerous the morning when a fire alarm went off at the hotel we were staying at. Our room was up on the fourth floor. This wasn't a problem for us, since we could just take the elevator up and down, until there was an emergency and we had no way out other than four flights of stairs. Matt ended up running down the stairs, with the wheelchair in hand, while I tried to slowly make my way down the stairs with Harper. After a couple flights, I became extremely lightheaded, so I ended up scooting down until Matt was able to return and help me.

Luckily, there wasn't actually a fire. Someone had pulled the alarm. But had it been an actual emergency, we would've been in trouble. Now, if I can't get a room on the ground floor, I always talk to reception about what their evacuation plan is for disabled people should an emergency arise. During a recent hotel trip, the woman behind the counter went on a scavenger hunt to find someone who would have an answer. They never found one, so instead they said that, in the event of an emergency, I should call down to the front desk and someone will come up to help me. Surely, you can see how many holes are in that plan.

This is why I scoff when someone tells me that profits are what will drive businesses to be accessible. Of course it won't. If businesses have gone this long without adapting, chances are pretty slim that they will suddenly decide that they can't stand to lose that small bit of profits. Often, these places get away with being inaccessible, simply because we don't have any other options.

Which brings me to the most important point, in my opinion:

Third, we are human beings, not dollar signs. An argument founded on saving money in the name of discrimination will absolutely never make sense to me. It's incredibly dehumanizing to tell disabled people that their right to exist in the world is less important than your profit margins. Because, that is truly what is at risk here. It's not about disabled people being denied access to one or two places and just going to the places that are accessible. It's about us being denied access, especially full access, to the majority of places we try to go to. What it truly comes down to is whether or not you believe disabled people have a right to exist in this world.

Denying us access is denying us the right to exist.

NOT DIFFERENTLY ABLED

Have you ever been told, "The only real disability is a bad attitude?" Or, the ridiculously patronizing, "You're not disabled, you're differently abled?" Or, how about, "you're only disabled if you let yourself think that way?" Perhaps you are someone who has once said these things to someone. If you are, stop now and let me explain to you why those phrases aren't actually helping disabled people, but how they are hurting us instead.

Here's the thing, "disabled" is not a bad word and refusing to acknowledge my disability doesn't help me or anyone else with a disability. **I know that may be hard to believe for some people, but it's true.** Allow me to explain all the ways this attitude is harmful to disabled people:

1. Denying Accessibility

As we've just discussed, it's incredibly important for disabled people to have access to public, and even private, places. We want our friends and family to choose places that are accessible to us for outings and events, if they really want us to be there, that is. If truly the only disability is a bad attitude, then making places accessible for those with disabilities could be seen as enabling that bad attitude. For instance, when I'm faced with a few steps on a bad day and someone says, "Come on, it's only a couple of steps, you can do it. Stop being so negative and believe in yourself." Sure, I could push myself to climb those few steps, but it takes far more energy than any able bodied person could ever imagine. Me climbing the stairs isn't some inspirational moment of me overcoming my disability, it's me inflicting more harm and pain on my body than is necessary for the comfort of an abled person.

Disabled people don't need to overcome our disabilities to better fit into the abled world around us, yet, that is what we are constantly told. The fable of the disabled person "overcoming" their disability by becoming, or acting, more abled is celebrated over and over again. It's constantly spread because it gives abled people an excuse to stop making the world more accessible to us. Abled people make themselves feel better about denying us this accessibility, because they are "helping" us, and disabled people get gas-lighted into believing that maybe we really don't deserve accessibility.

I once had a discussion with a fellow disabled person who told me that we shouldn't expect anyone to make things accessible to us. She even went as far as to say that asking for accessibility was asking for the world to revolve around us. The internalized ableism is strong in that one.

We aren't divas or high maintenance for asking for accessibility. We don't have "special needs." We have the same needs as every other human, they're just met in different ways. We need food, education, entertainment, work, and all the other things that able bodied people need. That's why it doesn't make any sense to deny us that same access simply because the access itself looks different.

2. Blame

It's ok if abled people deny us access, because our disabilities are really just a state of mind that we refuse to break free of. In other words, it's our fault that we're still disabled, because we haven't chosen to let go of that mentality. This seems to be especially true with invisible disabilities and illnesses, since people tend to think that if we don't look a certain way, then we couldn't possibly be as ill or disabled as we say we are. I have had countless abled people tell me that I just need some fresh air or to think optimistically to get rid of my PTSD, anxiety, and depression. Life isn't like Peter Pan, a little pixie dust and happy thoughts won't make our disabilities suddenly disappear. Nor would many of us want it to.

Blaming disabled and/or chronically ill people for their disabilities/illnesses doesn't help us to get magically better. It's not like a powerful speech given by a coach in a sports movie that inspires the team to play harder and win. No, this "if you just tried harder" attitude isn't about disabled people at all. It's about abled people. It's about excusing their refusal to adapt and giving them a false sense of control over their future as abled/healthy people. After all, if disabilities are really just a state of mind that we can think away, then abled people don't have to face the reality that they, too, can become disabled at any moment.

Using us to make people feel better about their abledness not only doesn't actually protect them from becoming disabled, it's also incredibly harmful to the self-esteem of disabled people. When I'm stuck in a depressive episode, having someone tell me that I'm sad because I'm choosing to be sad doesn't make the sadness go away. It makes it worse. Because now I not only feel depressed, I also have overwhelming guilt about my depression and wonder why I can't just snap out of it. Blame doesn't inspire us to rise up out of our disabilities, *because we aren't faking our disabilities*. Our needs are quite real and can't simply be wished away.

3. Disabilities Aren't Inherently Bad

You know what makes life with a disability hard? Ableism. I know, I know, I've said that before, but that's because it is so important for people to understand. Living in a world that values people based on their productivity, that is widely inaccessible, and that constantly looks down on disabled people as being "less than" is the absolute most difficult part of my disability that I've encountered.

Being told that you are a burden to society carries a weight like no other. It wraps its cold hard grip around you, squeezing your breath out, and dragging you down into the depths of depression. It leaves you questioning everything, including if there is any purpose in you continuing to live in this world when the world has made it so clear that there is no place for you in it.

Now, I know that this subject can be tricky when talking about chronic illness, as many of us would wish our illnesses away, if possible. But, it's important to recognize the distinction between hating my illnesses, and hating my disability. Yes, I hate that I can't dance without passing out, or that my life has become about conserving spoons. But I don't hate that I'm disabled, not anymore at least. I've learned that there is no shame in using mobility aids, or having a disability placard, or asking for accessibility. I'm not embarrassed to say that I'm disabled, or that I have chronic illness. Yes, I hate many of the symptoms I deal with, but not my disability itself.

I'll sometimes find myself anxious about using my mobility aids or wearing my compression socks in public. It's not because I think I don't need them, or that I think they're something that should be hidden. I feel anxious because of how the majority of the abled world views my devices and unusual clothing. I hate the judgmental, pitying, and quizzical looks. Strangers staring at me as I go about my day tends to make me a little self-conscious.

No, most disabled people don't hate their disabilities. Yet, many abled people seem to hate us, just for existing. They promote ideas of eugenics when it comes to preventing disabled babies from being born. The idea of weeding out any 'undesirable' trait in utero is lauded as great medical progress. I've heard even staunch "pro-lifers" celebrate abortion if the fetus has a disability. It's seen as an act of mercy, since the life of a disabled person isn't viewed as worth living.

A good portion of the anti-vaccine movement is based on ableism and the idea that all disabilities are tragic. I've watched parents scream and protest life-saving medicine on the unsupported fear that it would make their child neurologically different. It seems there are people who would rather their child die of the Measles than be Autistic. Not that there is any actual evidence whatsoever of a correlation between vaccines and Autism, anyway.

There are multiple supposedly romantic movies and TV shows that depict a disabled person putting their life at risk to be with someone or do one big thing…like go to a concert. Their inevitable death is then portrayed as beautiful and happy because obviously that concert is the best thing that could've ever happened to a disabled person, and is totally worth dying for.

Maybe the typical abled person isn't as extreme as those described above, but denying my disability or treating it like it's a dirty word sends me the exact same message. It tells me that they believe my disability is something I should be ashamed of, that it's a tragedy, and that I should try harder to be abled once again or die trying. It tells me that the person saying these things is uncomfortable with who I am, and that they believe I should be as well. It tells me that they think that their abled-ness makes them more of an authority on my experiences and identifiers than I am. And, it tells me that they think my life doesn't have value.

Some people may think that I'm over exaggerating. That this word can't possibly have that much power. And I'm sure that a good portion of the people who are so afraid to use the word "disabled" don't want to see all disabled people die. But, ableism is harmful even when it's done with good intentions. Benevolent ableism still kills.

You see, most of these things don't start with "Death to all disabled people!!" They start with "Don't call yourself disabled, that's so negative." It starts with an assumption that disability is a bad thing so it should be glossed over or sugar coated, as if the word itself is an insult. People will say that they are trying to humanize disabled people by calling us "differently abled" or some other euphemism. They don't seem to realize that we don't need them to humanize us because we're *already* human. This belief that we're somehow subhuman is what leads to the deadly side of ableism.

I urge everyone to say the word. Call me disabled. Refer to anyone who refers to themselves as disabled, as...well...disabled. Recognize that if you're struggling to say the word, then perhaps you have some prejudices and biases that you need to reflect on and move past. If you're a disabled person, know that it's not your job to make abled people feel more comfortable with who you are.

I'm a disabled woman, and there is nothing wrong with that.

Part Four

TIPS & TRICKS

A SPOONIE WEDDING

It finally happened!! After years of waiting, on January 2nd, 2018 I married the love of my life. After a very short engagement, we celebrated our union with our dream wedding...well, as close to our dreams that we could get on a small budget and limited supply of spoons. Honestly, though, it couldn't have been more perfect.

I was nervous leading up to the wedding, not because I was unsure of committing myself to him, but because I wasn't sure how I'd get through the day with POTS and EDS. I can barely leave the house without quickly being overwhelmed by fatigue, so how was I supposed to get through two days of activities, socializing, decorating, and more? And what about the cost? Money is tight with me not being able to work full-time, so how do we make sure we have everything we want without going into debt?

Well, lucky for you, I'm an avid researcher! I read multiple blogs on cutting wedding costs and asked for advice from fellow spoonies who've had weddings. I combed through hundreds of reviews for different products and companies, trying to find the best bang for our buck. In the end, we were able to have a beautiful wedding and romantic honeymoon on a budget of $2,500, and I was able to enjoy every minute of it!

Everyone's dream wedding is personal and unique, so you may not use the same things that we used, but I've learned a few tricks through my past wedding experiences (Maid of Honor three times, baby!) and diligent researching that I think anyone could benefit from.

1. Marry your best friend

This is good advice whether you have chronic illnesses or not. Before I started dating Matt, I thought that the whole "my husband is my best friend" thing was just a lie people would tell to make their spouses feel better. Now I know that it is not only possible, but preferable as well.

I know I've bragged about him a lot, so just bear with me for a little longer. He makes me laugh harder than anyone else in this world. I am never more myself than when I'm with him. There's no pretense, no need to hide parts of myself away. I get to be the raw pure me and he loves me still.

I'm sharing all of this so that you know that love like this exists. I didn't feel any of these things in my previous relationships and thought that this kind of love was pure fantasy. It's not. If you don't feel comfortable enough with someone to be seen without makeup, in your old sweats that are falling apart, and Oreo crumbs littered on your shirt (or whatever your "natural" state looks like), then maybe wait a bit to get married. I find this to be especially important when you have chronic illnesses, as there are days where I can barely get out of bed, let alone bathe. Let me tell you, your relationship reaches a new level of comfort when they have to help you onto a hospital toilet or carry a cup of your urine for testing. You want someone you trust by your side through it all.

2. Keep it small

This is a good tip for both budget and spoonie friendly weddings. We'd contemplated eloping, but eventually decided that we wanted to spend our special day with those closest to us. Our guest list ended up being only 55 people, around 30 of which were actually able to attend. It can certainly be challenging to keep a guest list that small, but for us it was absolutely necessary. It made the whole day more intimate and with a lot less pressure. I didn't worry about having to explain to my great-aunt's nephew's cousin about why I had a wheelchair but could also walk, nor did I have to spend the whole evening going around to greet hundreds of people individually.

It was small, and it was perfect for us. It was also perfect for our budget.

For every guest, you have to account for food, desserts, chairs, tables, drinks, etc. It all adds up quickly. Having fewer guests allowed us to afford more food, even sending guests home with doggie bags. Everyone had their fair share with plenty left over. We even got to all sit at one U shaped table together! And, because everyone there was someone close to us, they were all more than willing to help switch decorations, put out food, and break everything down at the end of the night.

Keeping our wedding party small was also a huge help. For every bridesmaid, groomsman, or other attendant you have to get gifts, flower arrangements, and other accessories. You have more schedules to work around, events to plan, and rehearsing. We cut down on all of that by having one attendant for each of us, each choosing our oldest and dearest friend. All our other friends and family who would've been attendants were still at the wedding and helped out wherever they could, so they were very much an active part of our union, just without buying the dress or renting the tux.

3. Search for bargains

My dad instilled in me the habit of comparing products and reading reviews before buying anything. This was a skill I got a lot of use out of when planning our wedding. People love to say "You get what you pay for" to imply that things that cost less aren't always the best quality, but I've found that to not always be true. Not if you research it enough.

Our wedding venue was at least half the cost of every other venue in town, and yet it was beautiful, quaint, and accommodating. For less than $150, we paid for our small wedding cake and mini cupcakes for all the guests (with lots of leftovers!). Our food cost under $400, and was super easy to order through a catering website. Nearly all of our decorations were ordered off of Amazon and they were all of great quality.

Perhaps the best bargain of all was my wedding dress. Every bride knows that wedding gowns cost a small fortune, which is infuriating since you only get to wear them once. I was nervous to order my gown online, but knew that I had to, as going into the shop to try on several dresses would be too much for me at the time. After reading a ridiculous number of reviews, I found my dream dress on Amazon for $125. That was with custom measurements and added sleeves. The best part? It in no way looked or felt like a cheap dress. I received a multitude of compliments on it, and I don't think I could have loved any dress any more than this one.

Higher cost doesn't always equal higher quality. A little research can end up saving you tons of money in the long run.

4. Get creative

Weddings are a huge industry in the US. Places that are dedicated to weddings cost a ton, therefore it can pay to stray from the traditional path when it comes to your wedding. We got married on a Tuesday, which automatically cut our already fairly affordable venue costs in half. A creative friend of mine looked up how to make floral arrangements and ended up making all of our bouquets, boutonnieres, and centerpieces with a mix of flowers ordered online and some bought at a grocery store. Matt's brother officiated the ceremony. One of his sisters, who does photography as a hobby, took all of our photos. My Matron of Honor painted our guest book. We served gourmet pizzas for a fraction of other catering costs. I did my own nails. We broke away from many of the typical wedding costs, yet still had a wonderful event that showed off our personalities.

Look for areas that you can cut out costs. We didn't give out favors to the guests because we figured the dinner, desserts, and drinks kinda count as guest favors. I doubt a little tiny bag of candy would make our guests feel more appreciated than the rest of the food served. Don't get everything monogrammed or personalized. I have been to many weddings and not once did I pay attention to whether or not their napkins had the couples' initials on them. Fancy linens, expensive serving platters, personalized everything, on and on. All of those are areas that soak up funds fast but aren't truly needed.

Getting creative helps for your chronic illness, as well. We put tall chairs with decorative bows at the altar so that we could sit during the ceremony. I wore compression tights as well as an abdominal binder. There were plenty of electrolyte drinks at the site and never a shortage of places for me to sit whenever needed. The cold January temperatures helped with my vasoconstriction, which meant I was less dizzy and able to do more than usual. Having our wedding on a week day allowed me to rest up for the rest of the week before our honeymoon over the weekend. Even the time of year was budget friendly, since prices are always better during the off-season.

Not everyone will have someone capable of doing flowers, photography, officiating, or whatever, but I believe everyone has someone capable of something creative. Maybe your friend dabbles in baking and can bake you a cutting cake? Or perhaps you know a seamstress who can sew you a completely original dress? Or you might have a friend with a gorgeous garden full of flowers that they are willing to share with you? Now, understand that not everyone is able or willing to give away their talent and skills for free (particularly if they are professionals in their field), but sometimes they are in a position to offer a discounted price as a wedding present to you. Get creative and think outside the box, it will save you a fortune in the end.

5. Choose your people wisely

Wedding preparation is incredibly hectic, even without chronic illnesses thrown in! Many brides and grooms talk about feeling frazzled all day, getting dizzy from not eating, or being too exhausted to enjoy any of it. Choosing who you surround yourself with on the day can make a huge difference. Every spoonie bride and groom needs a supportive team that is willing and able to help in any way possible.

I was incredibly lucky in this department. The day before the wedding, when decorating the chapel, I could barely string two words together because my brain was so overloaded. The most helpful people were ones who came in, got a general idea of what I wanted, and then ran with it. They made it all come together wonderfully without asking me to stand over them directing every move. My Matron of Honor brought a bag of survival items to keep me well hydrated and salted throughout the day. My mother-in-law arrived early to finish decorating while my sister-in-law was doing my hair and makeup. And all our wonderful guests helped change over decorations, take pictures, or anything else that was needing to be done.

I'm not being hyperbolic when I say that I couldn't have gotten through the day without my team supporting me and I don't think I would've had nearly as good of a time if I was busy worrying about impressing everyone or playing the good hostess. Keep toxic people as distant from yourself as possible. If you have someone in your life who can't go a day without bombarding you with criticism, they don't really need to be spending a lot of one on one time with you on your wedding day, if they're there at all. You need to feel safe and secure or else all your energy gets burned up just by being in fight or flight mode. I felt incredibly at ease the entire day of my wedding because I was surrounded by so much love and support. It truly made such a big difference.

6. Accept the help that's offered

Choosing your people wisely doesn't work if you don't actually accept the help your people offer. Many of us, myself included, are reluctant to ask for help because we don't want to feel like burdens. But, we aren't burdens. The people who love you want to help you, and it's ok to accept help. It doesn't make you weak or needy, it just makes you human. If you try to do it all on your own, you will likely end up overextending yourself before the ceremony has even begun. So, unless you can afford to pay for people to take care of everything, you will need help and shouldn't be afraid to ask for it.

I've always struggled with accepting help because I felt like I should be able to do it all on my own. Truthfully, I might have been able to do it on my own, but if I had, I know I wouldn't have had the energy to walk down the aisle, or enjoy our first dance. And those who helped me knew that, as well. They were all excited being able to help us get married, and it made everything just a little more special because so much love went into all of it. Accept help. Be gracious, of course, but accept the help. It will make all the difference.

Remember, at the end of the day the thing that should matter more than anything else is that you and your loved one are married. Weddings are beautiful and fun, but they are nice additions to a marriage, not the main ingredient. Don't put so much pressure on yourself, or the day, to be perfect in every way. Don't think about what others think or if they are judging you. I assure you, we got plenty of funny looks for getting married on a Tuesday, serving pizza, and doing our own flowers, but none of that mattered. Matt said it best, when talking about a few critical glances we received, "I'm not marrying them, I'm marrying you. So I don't care what they think of our wedding, as long as we're happy with it." Focus the majority of your energy on your health and your partner; the rest is just icing on the very expensive cake.

WHEN A SPOONIE TRAVELS

Before POTS changed my life, I loved to travel. Spontaneous trips were a favorite of mine, just picking a location and driving off for a weekend, discovering all this place had to offer once I got there. The most thought that I put into what hotel to stay at was to look for safe parts of town, but I loved to find unique hotels off the beaten path. Flying is a great way to get somewhere fast, but I was partial to the philosophy that the destination is only half the fun, getting there is just as exciting.

However, once POTS came on the scene, traveling even a short distance became a whole lot more complicated...but not entirely impossible. I've taken a few small trips since becoming disabled, and one big one to the happiest place on Earth, so I thought I would share with my fellow spoonies some of the tips I've learned through mistakes, mishaps, and occasional smooth sailing.

It is important to note that everyone is affected differently by their chronic illnesses and/or disabilities, so not all of my tips will work for everyone. I will try to make them as general as possible, but also recognize that some things that are problems for me may not be a problem for you, and vice versa.

1. Bring someone you trust

Just to be clear, a disabled or chronically ill person absolutely should be able to travel alone if they so choose. Before POTS, I used to love solo trips. I'm lucky because I prefer to travel with Matt anyway, but if I didn't, I know my small amount of traveling would be pretty much impossible. Yes, some of that is due to my specific symptoms and needs, but the majority of it has to do with the lack of accessibility we have in our world. Trying to travel with a disability has only highlighted the accessibility issues we have. We should absolutely keep pushing for more accessibility and to make it easier for disabled people to travel on our own, but while that battle rages on, I think it's good to know that it'll help you a lot to have someone you trust with you on a trip.

I say someone you trust because you need to know that they will be nearby or come when you call them, if needed. Knowing that they have your best interest in mind helps as well, since they can serve as another pair of eyes looking out for accessibility or possible triggers around you. And, they are more likely to fight just as hard as you will to make sure that you enjoy the trip as much as they do.

Matt and I function as a team, and vacationing is no different. In our recent trip to Disney World, it helped me tremendously to know he was there with me and had my back. He pushed me in my chair around the park and could help navigate around large crowds or groups of people, since his perspective allowed him to see more than just other guests' butts (not a glamorous view). He could check out a ride to see if I could go on it while I sat in my chair in the shade. He could find foods for me that I could eat at the buffet, an inherently inaccessible way of dining. He knows my symptoms well, so it was like having two of me looking out for my needs, which helped tremendously. So, wherever you go, I highly suggest bringing along someone you know and trust who can help make the trip as spoonie friendly as possible.

2. Plan ahead but be flexible

I know that sounds completely contradictory, but it's a truth that us spoonies live with daily. Even when just going to a local event, I have to plan for when I take my meds, how much I need, how I'll get there, how I'll get back, what happens if I can't eat any of the food, what happens if I suddenly flare up, on and on. But, I also know that things can change at any moment, so I have to be willing to toss my plans out at some point, or to at least plan room for flexibility.

What does planning ahead entail for a spoonie? Well, obviously it's different for everyone, but some good general ideas are:

- prescriptions are filled ahead of time
- know how your mobility devices will be transported
- know how *you* will be transported
- reserve an accessible room at your hotel, if needed
- know where snacks, hydration, and meals will come from or if you'll have access to them
- make sure your party is aware of your accessibility needs
- know how you can get back to your room should you flare up while out (who will take you? what transportation would be needed? etc)

Having a plan outlined before you depart will help you to optimize your trip. You certainly don't want to be in the middle of a major flare and trying to coordinate how you'll get back to your room so that you can rest. Nor do you want to suddenly find yourself in need of a snack, but nowhere near where a snack can be found. And you definitely don't want to run out of your meds while you're on your vacation!

3. Research

Along with planning ahead is the research you need to do to help you plan. What do you need to research? Whatever you can! But, most importantly, research the accessibility of your destination. In doing research for our upcoming honeymoon, I ran across a couple of beautiful historic hotels I would have loved to stay at, until I discovered that they weren't accessible. They absolutely should be, and complaints need to be filed against them, but I'm so glad that I found out before and not after I sank a bunch of money into their establishment and sat through a four hour car ride to get there.

Finding out how accessible a place is isn't always easy. We've certainly gone to places that claim to be accessible and then, once we get there, we find out just how limited that access is. Disabled people looking to go to Disney World will read many reviews about how incredibly accessible they are, which is mostly true; however a good portion of their rides require a transfer from a wheelchair to the ride and would be difficult, if not impossible, for certain people. That's the kind of stuff that is good to know before you pay for an amazing vacation that you may not actually be able to enjoy.

4. Don't pack light

It might seem a little counter-intuitive, I mean, if you already have to make room for a mobility device, it could be difficult to find room for several bags as well. Yet, I've found it to be worth it. Even if we're going on a short day trip out of town, I pack more than I may need just to be sure I'm not caught unawares. Using a backpack instead of a purse has helped me a lot with this venture.

Your specific symptoms and needs will dictate what exactly you need to bring with you. My method of deciding is to think about what I would need for a normal day and what I would need for a bad flare, and then bring both. Extra medications, clothing that I can layer for temperature changes, sunglasses, noise cancelling earmuffs, emergency snacks, heating pads, blankets, OTC medication, and anything else I may think I'll need depending on the duration of the trip as well as the location. Yes, having extra luggage can be a pain, and often you don't end up needing half of the things you packed, but I've yet to regret over-packing for any trip I've gone on. It tends to be the item I think I'll need the least that I end up using the most.

5. Take breaks

Maybe this seems like a no-brainer, but I think it's important to state anyway. Especially when paying money to go on a spectacular vacation, we can feel pressured to try and do it all. Resting is like wasted money, or wasted time where you could be having fun with your loved ones. Yet, taking time to rest is absolutely imperative. If you don't, your body will eventually decide to force you into taking a break, which will end with you in a full blown flare having to miss out on more than just the vacation.

Plan ahead for breaks, but also know that you may need to take an unscheduled break because our bodies don't tend to follow our own schedules. I typically plan for resting the night we arrive, to try and recover from the trip there. I also plan only a couple events each day so that we don't have to rush and can take long breaks in between activities. And, should you end up feeling a flair coming on, go ahead and take a break even if it's not scheduled. Don't worry about missing an activity or so. You need to take care of yourself, even on vacation.

6. Remember Murphy's Law

You know Murphy's Law, right? The one that says "Whatever can go wrong, will go wrong?" It's an important part of any spoonie's vacation plan. Plan for emergencies, and ask your hotel what their plan is for evacuating disabled people should a crisis happen. You don't want to end up stuck at the top of the stairs when the fire alarm is blaring, unsure of how to get all the way down. It happens.

Know your exits, at all times. Know your emergency plans. Know the best way in and out of a place. Know what to do in the event of a flair up, including knowing where the nearest first aid center, urgent care, or hospital are located. It seems negative to approach your vacation plans with the idea of everything going wrong, and chances are good that most things will be fine, but having a plan for "just in case" can prove to be incredibly valuable for you and your loved ones.

7. Share your experience and leave reviews

You know what would make planning a vacation a lot easier? If every place was really open about their accessibility policies. Unfortunately, I've found that very few are. Many places will mark themselves as fully accessible only for you to find out that their idea of "accessible" is incredibly limited. Unfortunately, because of this, we can't always rely on a business' word in deciding if a place is truly accessible or not.

So, how do we find out then? Well, that's where I ask that every single person with chronic illnesses and/or disabilities tries to speak out about their experiences with a specific place or business. Leave reviews on their sites or on popular travel websites that share your opinion on just how accessible a place may be. Write blog posts, if possible, or even just share on social media (also a good place to leave reviews). I tend to scour the reviews of any particular place for mention of disability accessibility, but often I come up empty handed. When I see one, then I feel more comfortable with my decision to either go or stay away from a particular attraction or business.

Be vocal. Share your stories. Help other spoonies and disabled people find out what business are worthy of their patronage and which ones aren't. It can make a huge difference in the lives of many people.

Even with all these preparations, traveling with chronic illnesses or disabilities is hardly easy. Unexpected things pop up all the time. But, I've found that by doing these things I've been able to decrease the bad stuff and increase my fun, and I hope that they can help you, too.

TOXIC HOLIDAYS

For many people, the holiday season is full of excitement over the time they get to spend with all of their loved ones. For some, it creates a tinge of anxiety or panic as they think about seeing their racist uncle or the aunt who always asks when they're going to get pregnant. And then there are some who are either alone for the holidays, or feel alone as they are surrounded by a toxic family.

What is a toxic family? Toxic doesn't mean they're all drenched in radioactive materials. It's more like they themselves sort of exude radioactivity, making everyone around them feel slowly worse and worse as time goes on. Toxic relationships are unhealthy relationships, typically based on mental, physical, verbal, or emotional abuse. In most toxic relationships, the abusive person uses manipulation, belittling, and other such tactics in order to make the other person feel as useless and small as they possibly can. Sounds like a recipe for a truly exciting holiday dinner, doesn't it?

Cutting ties with a toxic family or toxic family members is far more difficult than most people imagine. If it's the family you grew up in, then that's the only family you've ever really known, how can you just walk away from that? If you married into a toxic family and your partner isn't ready to cut ties with them, then how could you possibly avoid them and just leave your partner to deal with the pain? But, truly, I believe one of the things that makes it so difficult for people to walk away from a family that constantly abuses them, is the way this type of dynamic is portrayed as acceptable in entertainment of all kinds.

Pretty much every single TV show, book, and movie I've ever seen that depicts a toxic family relationship has a story that's presented as such: the person trying to distance themselves from the family are selfish jerks, the abusive family members have some good qualities which supposedly makes up for all the pain they cause, and in the end the one who was trying to create healthy boundaries decides to accept their family as "quirky" and the cycle of abuse just continues. These movies are especially prevalent around the holidays or are often movies with holiday themes. Seriously, think about it and you'll be shocked.

Anyway, my point is not to dive into the analysis of the entertainment industry's obsession with glorifying unhealthy relationships, as worthy a topic that is. Rather, I want to help people with toxic families break away from that normalizing behavior and find ways to keep their holidays cheery and bright.

1. You don't have to go

Maybe this one seems obvious, but I know plenty of people who are terrified of the holidays because they feel obligated to go home and spend time with their toxic families. Many spoonies worry about having to face the family members who refuse to believe the validity of their illnesses, no matter what the doctors say, and who regularly accuse them of being attention seekers. There are spoonies worried about getting drilled about jobs again, or being called lazy because they are on disability, or family members who scream about how they shouldn't be forced to pay for the spoonie's medical bills, whether directly or indirectly. All of these situations can be devastating.

I'm here to tell you that you're under no obligation to go. If it is possible to stay away (as it's not possible for all), then stay away. Yes, it's likely that you will have some kind of consequence from it, such as a major guilt trip and missing out on Grandma's famous mac & cheese, but the benefit of avoiding the yearly deep depression that follows the constant criticism and manipulation can certainly outweigh even the yummiest of meals.

Spending the holiday alone is often portrayed as sad and pathetic, but, for some, it's liberating. Make your favorite holiday dishes on your own and spend the day watching your favorite holiday movies and TV specials. Sounds like a winning combination to me! If you have a partner, understanding extended family, or kids of your own, you can make the holidays cheery in your own home surrounding yourself only with those who are loving and supportive. I truly believe that it is possible to make your own family, whether it's through friends, kids, a spouse, your spouse's family, or whatever...you can decide who you let into your life, so try to choose those who affect you in a positive way.

2. Boundaries, boundaries, boundaries

If you have no choice but to go, as some truly don't have a choice, then arm yourself against the onslaught of cruelty you know will be waiting for you. Creating a wall of strong boundaries between you and the toxic people in your life is a must! It's one of the best ways to protect yourself. Boundaries can take multiple different forms and vary from person to person and situation to situation. You get to decide what is right for you with your toxic family.

One relatively (pardon the pun) easy way of keeping a strong boundary is by following a "small-talk only, nothing personal" rule for all conversations. Sharing too much of your personal life with toxic people opens you up for hurtful criticism. Honestly, many toxic people will even turn small talk into an argument, but it's a lot less emotionally damaging for a toxic person to argue with you about whether or not the rain is beneficial than it is for them to argue about if you're wasting your life, a burden to society, or whatever other buttons they might push.

Typically honesty is my policy. I try to promote being courageously authentic, and not letting others determine how you live your life. However, I've also learned that not everyone deserves to see your authentic self. Not everyone deserves to be let into your life, even if they are the ones who gave you life to begin with. That doesn't mean you go in and lie or pretend to be someone else. Rather, you only show them the side of yourself reserved for acquaintances instead of baring your whole beautiful soul. Reserve your whole true self for those who have proven themselves worthy of seeing it.

3. Distractions

Another way to help avoid unnecessary hurtful conversations is to load yourself up with distractions to keep busy. Bring a supportive friend, your kick-ass spouse, or even just a book you love. You can keep yourself occupied by chatting with your friend or spouse, or keep your nose buried in your favorite story of far off places. You could even bring this book! No matter the type of distraction you bring, it's helping you close yourself off to harmful conversations.

It's important, however, that anyone you bring for support understands the situation and are prepared to help you through it. If you bring someone who is unaware, they may end up adding to the stress of the day as they can't comprehend why you're talking so little with your family.

There are lots of easy ways to create distractions for yourself. You can text a friend throughout the day, if you are stuck on your own. Suggest watching a holiday movie, which can keep most of the family occupied and less inclined to talk. Hang out with any family members that aren't toxic, children are often great for this. People are less likely to bother you about being distant when they see you playing with the kids. No matter how you go about it, having a distraction that you can immerse yourself in can help you to avoid feeling trapped and helpless around your toxic family.

No matter what you do, remember that it's okay to protect yourself and your mental health. You're not obligated to open yourself up to toxic people or to share any part of yourself with them. Toxic people have a way of convincing you that you owe them everything, but you don't. You don't owe them your time, your sanity, your joy, or any part of your life. And you don't owe them an explanation as to why.

Remember, the holidays are for you as well, and you deserve to celebrate them however you would like.

DON'T GIVE UP

Don't give up. Words that we often hear muttered by strangers who aren't sure what to say, or family who miss who you were before you got sick, or friends who don't understand, or doctors who are looking for a way to end an awkward conversation. You know the conversation I'm talking about, the one where you're crying because every aspect of your life has changed but no one can give you any answers on how to get back to where you were. The conversation where you struggle to get the words out or string a sentence together because your body is shaking with the heaving sobs. It's the conversation that everyone diagnosed with an incurable chronic illness has at some point, in some form, because how can you not, when receiving a lifetime diagnosis of an incurable illness that will change everything about your world?

Don't give up, they assert, hoping it will appease you because they don't have any other words of advice to give. Don't give up, they sigh, wanting you to magically snap out of it through the power of thought and return to who they want you to be. Don't give up, they utter, because they are watching you seemingly fall apart and want more than anything to help hold you together. The intentions are usually good, and yet, the phrase bounces off of me as the voice in my head screams, "What other choice was I given?!" It shrieks at me as I try to hide the truth behind a smile, the truth that sometimes I *want* to give up.

I want to be fully honest with you all, so here I am, opening up my heart and bleeding onto the page. I have had so many people tell me that I inspire them with my positive attitude or my drive to keep fighting, but the truth is that there are many times when I don't want to fight. There are times when the anger and frustration I feel at being forced to fight every moment of my life aches and burns straight down to my bones. There are moments when I'm filled with bitter resentment at being given a life of endless struggle. I want to share all of this anger and agony with you, because I have a feeling that you, too, have days where you want to throw in the towel and stop fighting.

And, yet, what I want to tell you all more than anything in the world is: "Don't give up." Before dismissing me as a hypocrite and brushing my words off as another empty gesture, know that when I tell you "don't give up," I say it with the complete understanding that "giving up" looks different for every single person. Hell, it looks different to me depending on the situation, day, feelings, goals, or weather. So, when I say "don't give up" to you, I don't mean for you to cling onto being the way I think that you're supposed to be, a sub-textual meaning that often lingers behind those words as they are uttered by others who don't understand their impact. What I mean is don't give up on whatever you need to hold onto for that day, that minute, that fraction of a moment. Whatever it is you feel the urge to hold onto, hold onto it and don't give up.

When I first became disabled by my illnesses, I was told not to give up quite often by many different people. I heard it when I cut back my hours at work, when I got a wheelchair, and when I applied for disability. The general comment seemed to be telling me not to give up on being abled or healthy, to hold onto those things with all of my might. But, admitting I was disabled wasn't me giving up. In fact, it was freeing.

Accepting my body's limitations helped me to balance out what I was capable of doing each day, and to stop wasting my precious energy on things that didn't matter. For many abled people, admitting I was disabled was seen as admitting defeat, but for me, it was me choosing not to give up on the things I loved most in my life. Stepping back from the job I loved hurt. It felt as though a piece of me was ripped out, but it wasn't me giving up. It was me recognizing that I had a choice to either use my energy for work or have energy to be a mom, and I chose the latter. I chose not to give up.

So, don't give up. Even if all you can manage to force yourself to do is to keep breathing, do it. I have fought my way through days where it takes all the strength I have to go on existing. Not because I contemplate suicide, but because I get wrapped up in the fantasy of nonexistence. A misty dream of nothingness: no pain, no hurt, no tears, no sadness, and no guilt. Or days when the idea of growing old fills me with dread because I cannot begin to imagine how the regular wear and tear that comes with old age will mix with my EDS body that already begs for rest after the slightest amount of activity. Days when the uncertainty of the future hangs over me like my own personal rain cloud, and it takes everything I have just to keep pushing through the day, knowing it only brings me one day closer to the future I fear. Most people would look at me during those days and shake their heads, clicking their tongues while saying, "She just gave up" because they don't realize how much I'm fighting for every single breath I take.

There are so many different ways that I refuse to give up. There are days when I tackle each obstacle in front of me with a smile and bright optimism. There are stretches of weeks when I force my way through by writing even when I don't feel like it, or exercising even when my body aches, or going to see the friend I wanted to see, or throwing my daughter a birthday party, or simply making it out the front door. There are moments when I'm suddenly hit with a severe flare, where I literally drag myself from where I am to wherever it is I need to go, all the while breathing out the words "It's ok, you're ok, you can do this, just get to the bed, you're ok, you've got this," because that's the only way I know how to keep myself going. No, there is no one way to refuse to give up.

Don't give up. But, also, don't let anyone define what giving up means to you. Don't give up. And, don't chastise yourself for not living up to the standards of people who will never understand just how much of a warrior you are. It's not your job to inspire others with your story. It's more than enough to try to simply inspire yourself to keep going. Forgive yourself for the days when you want to give up. You aren't weak because you get tired of fighting, or for feeling angry at the world for denying you the life you'd hoped for. You're human.

Be kind to yourself. Be true to yourself. And, don't give up.

ABOUT THE AUTHOR

Saidee Wynn began her writing career (can you call it a 'career' if you don't get paid?) in 2017 with her blog 'Spoonie Warrior.' She has been awarded with the "Best Mommy Ever" Award, which her daughter assures her is real. She lives at home with her loving husband, spunky kid, lazy dog, and codependent cat.

95153637R00100

Made in the USA
Columbia, SC
07 May 2018